The Art & Science of
RATIONAL EATING

by
Albert Ellis, Ph.D.
Michael Abrams, Ph.D.
Lidia Dengelegi, Ph.D.

Barricade Books Inc.
Fort Lee, New Jersey

Published by Barricade Books Inc., 1530 Palisade Avenue,
Fort Lee, NJ 07024

Printed in the United States of America.

Library of Congress Cataloging-in-Publication Data

Ellis, Albert.
    The art & science of rational eating / Albert Ellis,
Michael Abrams, Lidia Dengelegi.
    Includes bibliographical references and index.
    ISBN 0-942637-60-7: $14.95
    1. Eating disorders—Popular works.   2. Rational-
emotive psychotherapy.   3. Cognitive therapy. I. Abrams,
Michael. II. Dengelegi, Lidia. III. Title. IV. Title: Art
and science of rational eating.
RC552.E18E44   1992   92-17733
616.85'260651—dc20   CIP

9   8   7   6   5   4   3   2

Contents

Introduction

Why can't I control my eating? Why am I fatter than I want to be? Why does it seem so hard for me to lose weight? Why can't I *keep* my weight down? Questions like these place you among the countless people who have agonized about their eating. As psychologists, we have worked with hundreds of people who have sought assistance with their weight and eating. And we have made the unstartling discovery that weight reduction has an extraordinarily low success rate. By answering the above questions and by offering psychological alternatives to dieting, we hope to relieve many anguished readers. How? By exploring four important areas.

First, we shall review current research that will give you the foundation of rational eating behavior. Second, we shall explore the process of self-understanding, to show how your disturbed feelings about eating can be traced to irrational, inflexible, absolutistic thinking. We will show how rigid, unscientific thinking leads to slips, failures, or even binges, and how learning to realistically evaluate situations and options will let you make your greatest single advance towards personal control. Third, we will present case studies of real people with various kinds of weight and eating problems, thus making your own difficulties strikingly apparent. Throughout this book are cases of actual clients who have succeeded, have failed, or have rationally accepted themselves without change.

Finally, we will present an effective psychological strategy to help you make the changes you may decide to pursue. Rational-emotive therapy (RET) will help you as the foundation for either choosing to change or to accept yourself as you are. RET methods will give you the tools to bring about dietary change—if that is your choice.

History and Background of Eating Problems

The title of this book implies two things. The first is that there are rational and irrational ways to eat. The second is that eating is a choice. The popular view is that rational people eat precisely what their bodies need to live well, and irrational people distort their bodies as a result of their pathological eating. We agree with this view, but with an important warning: healthy bodies come in all shapes and sizes. Rational eating means considering your body's special needs and tendencies, and finding a way to eat that keeps your body healthy, energetic, and as pleasing to the eye as feasible. Easily said—but the weight where you feel your best may not be the weight that looks best in the eyes of western society. The popular view, as well as the view of most diet gurus, is that human bodies are elastic and that you can easily control your shape if you have a standard amount of "willpower." This idea governs most diet treatments and techniques. This sentiment is so universally held, that it is difficult for most people to believe that it is almost universally false.

Health care treatment is often based on sound research and clinical experience. Not so with weight and eating care. Eating myths, which are almost universal, stem from our natural tendency to blame other people's poor behavior on them, and to blame our own on some unavoidable circumstances. Thus, if someone cuts you off while driving you will usually conclude that they are dangerous idiots. However, if you cut off someone, you might explain it as being the result of someone making you late, or something else beyond your control. Because the majority of people are not obese, they tend to assume that people who are overweight are innately weak. Thinner people readily judge fat people as deserving to be fat as a result of their overeating. A term like overweight has no independent meaning. William Bennett of the Harvard Medical School Health Letter noted[1,2] that "the term "overeating" means that the "overeater" is overweight. If eating behavior did not produce deposits of body fat, we could not call it overeating. Thus to say that people get fat because they overeat is no different from saying that the sun comes up because it is morning."

We will show that the actual evidence robustly points in another direction. It shows that there are many different types of people, all shapes, sizes, and styles, and obesity, rather than being symptom of neurosis, may say no more about a person than her height, hair color, or skin texture. There is significant evidence that fat people do not eat more than slender people.[3-6]

Recent advances in the study and treatment of eating disorders, paradoxically, have done a great deal to advance the popular myth that obesity stems from emotional disturbance. Researchers of eating disorders like anorexia (extreme weight loss due to self-starvation) and bulimia (controlling one's weight by vomiting) have shown that these conditions go with disturbance. Many researchers assign obesity in the same class with eating disorders, despite the strong evidence that it is very different. What's more, popular "wisdom" holds that everyone reacts the same way to food and that in order to grow fat one must eat much more than a slender person would. Fatness is also wrongly considered to be evidence of mental disease and addiction.

Judging a person's personality by her weight is not limited to the fat person. The unusually slender woman may be arbitrarily labeled as anorectic. Even if she is naturally thin, she is "known" to have withdrawn from the world and from her own ability to love. Her lean and hungry look is "seen" as stemming from her inability to accept the reality of her life. In general we are often biased against people who look different. But we view fat people with special disdain. Their looks are seen as "evidence" of deficient will and character. Supposedly, they eat for love, they sublimate their sexual desire by quenching their impulses with unremitting volleys of victuals; they hide within an abundant sheath of corpulent isolation.

Fat is a barrier, a bellicose statement to others that, to some, justifies hostility in kind. The world says to the fat person, "Your fatness is an affront to me, so we have the right to treat you as offensively as you appear." Fat is not merely viewed as another type of tissue, but as a diagnostic sign, a personal statement, and a measure of personality. Too little fat and we see you as being antisocial, fearful and sexless. Too much fat and we see you as slothful, stupid, and sexually hung up.

In this book we shall argue against these notions by showing that obesity stems more from genetic and biological than from neurotic roots, and that most personality traits "causing" obesity actually originate from people lambasting themselves for being fat. We will also make clear that most weight problems can be solved psychologically—but differently from what popular psychology suggests.

Rational-Emotive Therapy and Psychology

Rational-Emotive Therapy (RET) was founded by Albert Ellis[7] in 1955 as the first of today's cognitive-behavior therapies (CBT). Cognitive refers to all processes of thinking. RET, the most popular cognitive therapy used by practicing therapists, helps people improve upon their thinking, and thereby improve their behaviors and emotions.

How can cognition help you master an overwhelming desire to eat? It cannot by itself, but thinking properly can enable you to achieve three important goals: 1) accepting yourself with your eating or weight problems; 2) conquering your inappropriate feelings that can block you from dealing with these problems; and 3) setting wise eating goals.

Changing your thinking is something like, and can be importantly connected with, "conditioning" your behaviors. Let's review the basic principles of conditioning to illustrate how thoughts can be conditioned. During the early part of this century a Russian physiologist named Ivan Pavlov experimented with the digestive secretions of dogs. These dogs were fed by a tube that permitted their food to be placed directly into their digestive tracts, bypassing their mouths. Pavlov observed that after a short duration of such feeding the dogs would begin to salivate at the mere sight of the lab assistants who provided the dogs with their daily powdered meat. He proposed that an artificial reflex had been created—a "conditioned reflex" or a "conditioned response." This idea became the basis for an entire movement in American psychology called behaviorism.

After reading of Pavlov's results, the American psychologist John Watson noted that if we observe the stimuli preceding an animal's behavior and then study the behavior that follows these stimuli, we need do no more to understand psychology. This is the basis of radical behaviorism, with which Watson provided the tools for a new approach to human problems. This notion was further developed by B.F. Skinner, who optimistically suggested that every human problem can be solved by this conditioning. Skinner's views hold that we all start with random behaviors, and if a certain behavior is rewarded or reinforced, we will probably increase it. If it is not rewarded, we will decrease it. A negative reinforcer, in contrast, is an unpleasant event that, *when removed*, tends to increase a behavior. Thus, removing a tight shoe will encourage us to walk more. Skinner did not believe, however, that punishment is an effective long-term tool for changing behavior. His suggestion to help an overeater change would be to keep her from delicious food rather than to punish her every time she overeats. Traditional behaviorists like Skinner and Watson were only concerned with behavior, and believed that thought or cognition has little to do with causing or blocking it.

However, several psychologists showed that thinking and acting affect each other. For example, Ulric Neisser, who wrote the first text on cognitive psychology, suggested that instead of seeing the mind as a switching unit, we should view it as an information processing system that considers new information in light of previous information in memory, and decides upon a response. Other cognitive psychologists such as Julian Rotter, Albert Ellis and Richard Lazarus stress that the human personality affects our environment, and our environment influences our personality. We don't simply respond to stimuli we are exposed to but we consciously and unconsciously *choose* to approach those that we like and *choose* to avoid those that we don't wish to be around. We can also influence our own and others' responses by thinking and talking (to ourselves and to others) about our feelings and actions.

Cognitive therapy and RET show that we do not have to directly experience a stimulus to respond, but we can watch others and respond to a stimulus the way they do. This is called modeling. Cognitive psychologists reject Skinner's notion that behaviors are randomly emitted and then reinforced, believing instead that we learn to respond first, and then whether or not we continue to emit them is based on how much reinforcement we get. Therefore reward and punishment are not essential to learning new behavior—they may have an effect but only on the frequency of our response: *in fact, we can be motivated to perform an act if we observe someone else being rewarded for it, and we can even reinforce ourselves.* Thus, you can reinforce the behavior you wish to see in yourself with your own thoughts. I (AE) discovered that people largely —but not completely—bring about their own feelings and actions by their thinking. I read this in several ancient philosophers' writings—especially Epictetus and Marcus Aurelius—and I clearly saw it in my own clients from 1943 to 1955. I found that when these clients thought realistically, logically, and preferentially, they created appropriate, self-helping emotions and behaviors. And when they thought unrealistically, illogically, and rigidly, they felt and acted inappropriately, against their own interests. I saw this even when I practiced psychoanalysis for several years; and as I saw it more clearly I gave up psychoanalysis, created rational-emotive therapy (RET) in 1955, and have been practicing and teaching it ever since.

RET gives people facing adversity two main tools for relief. First, it shows them how to accept themselves unconditionally, no matter how poorly they are doing. RET rejects *self-worth* or *self-esteem*, because we achieve this "good" state by focusing on and measuring our positive characteristics. Self-acceptance means that we *fully* accept ourselves *with* our good and bad behavior. Yes, fully. Of course, all humans can benefit from some specific changes. But telling ourselves that we absolutely *must* act well to be *good people*, we actually hurt our chances for improvement. Psychologists like Carl Rogers and Albert Bandura have said that children need unconditional acceptance by their parents to grow into healthy adults. That certainly helps! As adults, too, we'd better afford ourselves the same privilege so that we may develop into the adults that we want to be.

RET also teaches people, especially problem eaters, to have high frustration tolerance—which means giving into our urges for immediate gratification (like eating and drinking) only when they do *not* lead to later difficulties (like poor nutrition and drunkeness).

RET and Eating

Changing one's weight or eating style has been shown to be a most difficult long-term behavioral goal. The obese individual has a far lesser chance of permanently becoming thin than the heroin addict has of becoming clean, the crack user becoming drug free, or the alcoholic staying dry. With such an imposing obstacle to clear, the dieter had better learn to accept himself as he is, prior to making a grand effort to become thin. A person prone to self-downing actually discourages himself from changing traits that he loathes. If one hates oneself, one tends to be particularly unmotivated to work at self-improvement. "If I am no good, how can 'rotten me' improve my rotten traits?" Rational-emotive therapy encourages self-acceptance, not merely self-*efficacy*, and not self-*esteem*. As noted above, both of those forms of self-rating work badly. To achieve self-esteem you have to *perform* well. To achieve self-efficacy you have to constantly do *better than others*. By definition then, self-esteem and self-efficacy require relative ratings. But self-*acceptance* means that you view yourself as a "worthy person" *whether or not* you have great accomplishments. You do not rate *you*, your personhood, and do not blame yourself for not being better than you are. Of course, you work to improve your acts and traits in order to enjoy yourself and increase your standing in life. But it is unreasonable to disparage yourself simply because you are not the way that you presumably *should* or *must* be.

RET also helps you unblock your blocked-up thinking, feeling and behaving. Your eating problems—including the lack of motivation, will-power and self-acceptance that go with them—result from irrational thinking and behaving. Even if your problems with weight are biologically based, there is as yet no effective medical treatment that will safely reduce body fat. So RET and CBT seem to offer the main effective approach to weight control.[8-12] With

RET, you will learn to challenge your irrational thoughts and change your inappropriate feelings that put you out of control. There is no method of dietary change that will, by itself, produce results. *You* are the doer—or undoer—of these best laid plans. In fact, virtually all popular diet plans can work if they are adhered to precisely. This book shows you how to change yourself to fit the plans.

THE CASE OF MARY ELLEN

Mary Ellen insisted that her family made her eat too much and weigh thirty-five pounds more than she wanted to weigh. First, they stuffed her during her childhood. Second, they lambasted her for avoiding her school work and, lately, for getting only office temporary jobs. Third, they argued so bitterly with each other all the time that they "drove" her to constant TV watching and overeating. Right?

No, wrong! As Mary Ellen discovered when she started to have RET sessions, all these things that were supposedly responsible for her fatness were A's or Activating Events that *preceded* but hardly *caused* her Cs (Consequences) of overeating and fatness. Her Bs (Beliefs about her A's) largely led to her Cs; and her Bs were *her* creations and *her* responsibility. Thus, as a child, she *told herself* "I *must* stuff myself to the gills because I *have to* win my parents' approval by doing so." She also *told herself*, later on, "My parents are right. I *am* no good for avoiding my school work and for getting only temporary office jobs." Finally, when her parents kept bitterly arguing with each other she *told herself*, "They *must* not fight like this! I *can't stand* it! I *have to* drive myself to constant TV watching and overeating to distract myself from this bedlam!"

When Mary Ellen took responsibility for her *own* irrational Beliefs (iBs) and her *own* Consequences (Cs) and when she went on to D (Disputing) her iBs, she was able to *stand* criticism, to *bear* her parents' fighting, and to stop most of her TV watching and overeating.

Obesity Defined

The definition of obesity is similar to that originated by a Supreme Court Justice—for obscenity. To paraphrase the justice: "I cannot define it, but I know it when I see it." Virtually all definitions of obesity are based on arbitrary judgments,[13-15] which largely arise from personal bias. The criteria for "overweight" are largely socially based and keep changing over the years. Throughout the last century insurance weight charts have mandated "ideal" weights which have always been at odds with the actual weights of most people.[16] If you are a "heavy person" who strives to move the reading on your scale closer to the insurance company ideal, you may be surprised to find that this standard is hardly a valid measure. These charts are based on a highly biased sample of people who have applied for life insurance and not on a random sample of the general population. It is doubtful that these "ideal" weights actually do promote longevity for everyone. As we will elaborate on in our chapter on health, "ideal" weights are probably not ideal for everyone.

According to the Merck Manual "a body weight 20% over that given in standard height/weight tables is arbitrarily considered obesity." Because most weight standards are themselves arbitrary, the term "obesity" is unscientific. Other measures of obesity do not merely go by weight. For example, body fat percentage has been used to determine obesity. This is superior to the standards based on size and weight because it gets to the core of the health issue—the fat. Professional football players or body-builders for example, are frequently overweight, but not overfat.

Unfortunately this body fat method too has a notable flaw in that there is no universal standard for the right amount of body fat. We would expect such a standard to be based on the amount of fat that impairs health. Unfortunately, no one agrees on an amount of fat that is unhealthy. In fact, some researchers have found that it is usually healthier to be slightly obese than it is to be slightly undernourished. What's more, a complete absence of body fat is *fatal*, a fact that might surprise those thinness enthusiasts who refer to fat as though it is a disease.

Other definitions of "obesity" have similar flaws. The term "fat" is a judgment indicating "too much" body fat, while "overweight" means that a person exceeds some medical or statistical standard for "normal" weight. We have no consistent meaning for any of these terms.

Treatment

Throughout their long history, the various remedies for weight problems have met with poor outcomes at best. [17-21] Bennett, in his excellent historical review of twenty years of weight loss treatment found that the average loss in obesity treatment programs is between ten and twenty pounds. [2] And what a number of "remedies" there have been! These include: complete starvation, high fat menus without limit, spartan fare arranged in complicated time sequences, metabolic stimulants, central nervous system drugs, even psychoanalysis! All these and more have been tried to save the fat person from his body.

Yet, most people who restrict their intake fail to reach a desired body weight, and most people who achieve the "right" weight fail to stay there. Why? Largely because "obesity" has many different causes [22-25] which have been poorly understood by many of those treating this "malady." Body fat levels are a result of genetic, endocrinological, structural, societal, cognitive, and behavioral factors. What's more, despite the vast array of programs and methods, many authorities even challenge the idea that obesity is undesirable or worthy of formal treatment.[1,2,17,26,27] These researchers suggest that obesity treatment may actually be unethical, because its efficacy has never been demonstrated.[1,17]

However, despite the often dismal results obtained by most obesity treatment methods, people persistently seek out new and better ways to reduce their weight, and, over time, many do have some success. The issue of success itself raises problems because it is difficult to clearly define what success is. Many people lose a substantial amount of weight but fail to reach their goal, or the goal set for them by the weight charts or a health-care professional. Others reach, or exceed, their goals only to gain some or all of their weight back. We think that if we were to define dietary success as achieving target weight and maintaining it fairly precisely for several years, we would discover a very small percentage—about five percent—achieving it. Yet heavy persons keep searching for the cure to their affliction, which they rank among the major causes of suffering. It is something of a paradox that obesity is a major source of anguish in a world that has seen so much starvation. (But perhaps not. Obesity may be an evolutionary consequence of chronic starvation, an idea we will elaborate on in Chapter 3.)

Psychologist Natalie Allon observed[28] that our personal view of the "fat" person strongly influences our judgments about the causes of that person's weight problem. If we are biased against the fat person, we will tend to conclude that the obesity comes from his or her avaricious and indulgent nature. But if we take the point of view that obesity is largely a biological trait, we will view the fat person as just one who differs from other humans, only in fat content—not in character. Our bias against fat people has encouraged people to desperately seek, over and over again, a new way to end their suffering. Our society tells them that they can accept themselves only if they first change. Despite the popular view that fat people don't really try, many of them make sincere, sometimes extraordinary efforts to change their weights—with little or no luck! Our next case will illustrate this point.

THE CASE OF ARLENE

Arlene came to our office seeking relief from her 398 pounds. She was five feet two inches tall, and was thirty-nine years old. Her lowest weight, as an adult, was three hundred pounds, and even this was a result of one of her more successful diets. When asked about her treatment history for weight, Arlene told a story that seemed typical of very heavy women. Since her adolescence, she had sought help from literally dozens of physicians. Their remedies ranged from handing Arlene a standard exchange diet, and telling her to stick to it, to every fat reducing drug available. Each dietary regimen brought some hope of realizing her goal—to be "normal." Arlene repeatedly starved herself and drugged herself with the simple objective of having people stop making fun of her. She strongly disliked herself, not because of any action or omission on her part, but because others repeatedly reminded her of her problem.

She had given up hope of ever having a relationship, of going out on a date, of being loved by a man. The morning of her visit to the office she had taken a train that required her to pass through a turnstile, one that was designed for people of usual size. Determined to begin another treatment regimen for her weight she assertively pushed her way through only to feel her body wedge between the spokes and the wall of the device. The people behind her began to angrily urge her on. Arlene, with tears of rage, described that when the commuters around her realized that she was immobilized within the turnstile, several commuters began to laugh at her. Others got the attention of their companions so that they could point out this amusing oddity. She was stuck for several minutes before anyone offered to help. She did not cry though, nor give them the satisfaction of seeing that they could hurt her.

Despite her hardships, Arlene had worked at the same job for twenty-four years and was highly valued by her employer. She presented herself as an articulate, intelligent person who felt hurt by, but not vengeful towards, her detractors. Psychological testing included the Millon Clinical Multiaxal Inventory (MCMI), and the Minnesota Multiphasic Personality Inventory (MMPI). Her scores were essentially in the normal range with minor elevations on the Social Introversion and Hysteria scales on the MMPI, and higher than average on the Histrionic scale on the Millon. These are the scores of an individual who is upset about lacking affection and interpersonal contact. Her psychological profile indicated no pathology that would explain her weight.

She was placed on a very-low-calorie diet. This protocol included weekly medical examinations and weekly rational-emotive group therapy which stressed self-acceptance. She adhered with virtually no lapses. At one point, she persisted despite an entire month with no weight loss at all. Arlene ultimately lost 135 pounds over thirteen months.

Unfortunately she was still far heavier than she wanted to be, despite the fact that her diet included fewer than seven hundred calories per day. Her weight loss had declined to fewer than three pounds per month. Despairing, she told me (MA) that she could no longer sustain deprivation without results and went back to normal eating for a while. On a relatively ordinary diet she gained back sixty-five pounds in less than two months. At this point she made the decision that death would be better than the constant cycle of gains and losses and decided to risk surgery. She was operated on and received a bilio-pancreatic diversion. Fourteen months after surgery she weighed 255 pounds, no longer losing but satisfied that she could eat reasonably normally without being morbidly obese. With counseling and therapy she had learned to accept herself. She was still fat but realized that this is the way she was and probably would remain. Her main goal now is to make the most of her life.

Arlene was not a good candidate for psychological treatment for obesity. She tended to prove obesity researcher, Jules Hirsch's, statement: "The answer to obesity is to change societies' views of obesity." She was a rational person in an irrational world, which unfortunately would not accommodate her. It persisted in viewing her as weak, self-indulgent, stupid, or corrupt, depending on the values of the particular observer. RET helped Arlene despite this reality. It showed her that she could accept herself without requiring approval or acclaim from others. She came to understand that other people did not have the power to make her feel hurt or depressed, but that such feelings arose from her beliefs *about* their attitudes.

Many counselors, researchers, and physicians still have the same biases as lay people do. Heavy men, women and children seeking help are implicitly told that they must change if they are to be acceptable as human beings. RET says the opposite: all people, including fat ones, are to be unconditionally accepted as *persons*. Arlene was helped more by learning to accept herself in spite of her weight than she was helped by dietary or physical change.

Multiple Causes

Fatness, obesity, corpulence, overweight . . . as its many labels suggest, have many origins. When a slender person views a heavier person he tends to make judgments based on his own personal experience. Should he be the type that gains only slight weight after great amounts of food, he will tend to assume that obese people have to devour even more massive amounts to be as large as they are. This conclusion stems from the assumption that others' experiences are largely the same as our own. We will make clear in subsequent chapters that there are many fundamental physiological differences between fat and thin people. People without weight problems tend to assume that the fat person experiences hunger, taste, and satiety the same as they do. However, the research evidence strongly denies this position. The sensation of hunger is not a uniform experience, and varies within and among individuals.[29,30]

Given the stigma, physical discomfort, and social consequences of obesity, we can well conclude that most people do not want to be fat. Rather than assume that they maintain their fatness to slight the sensibilities of the slender person, or out of gluttony, we might parsimoniously conclude they *are* actually more hungry, or that for them food is more pleasurable and harder to resist. When we choose to believe that fatness simply results from excessive eating, we often "explain" why fat persons are so willing to eat themselves into a state of social isolation, pain, and moral repudiation by inventing that they have personality disorders. But, as we demonstrate, there is no evidence for this. The real explanation is that obesity is a complex phenomenon with many interacting causes.

The failure to fully appreciate this many-sided origin of obesity has made the poor outcome of most dietary programs much worse. It has also stopped the use of good methods to help reduce the anguish of people seeking to lose weight. Most treatments, instead, have stressed simple dieting procedures while ignoring the emotional and cognitive problems involved with dieting. Fat people are told that they must be disturbed because they need only eat "right." If they fail to employ such a simple solution they must be very crazy indeed. Unfortunately, among the many causes of weight problems, lack of will, sanity or character are often the least important. In what follows we shall show that information, appropriate thinking and appropriate feelings have far more to do with controlling weight and eating than any particular dietary approach. Yes, it is possible to lose substantial amounts of weight, but it requires hard work and clear thinking about the pros and cons of deciding to do so.

Notes to Introduction.

1. Bennett, 1984.
2. Bennett, 1987.
3. Stunkard, Coll, Lundquist & Meyers, 1980.
4. Coll, Meyer & Stunkard, 1979.
5. Meyer, Stunkard & Coll, 1980.
6. duBois, Goodman & Conway, 1989.
7. Ellis, 1962.
8. Stunkard, 1985.
9. Stunkard, Craighead & O'Brien, 1980.
10. Wadden, Sternberg, Letizia, Stunkard & Foster, 1989.
11. Schmidt, 1989.
12. Bennett, 1988.
13. Neggers, Stitt & Roseman, 1990.
14. Kraemer, Berkowitz & Hammer, 1990a.
15. Kraemer, Berkowitz & Hammer, 1990b.
16. Pollack-Seid, 1989.
17. Garner & Wooley, 1991.
18. Wooley & Wooley, 1985.
19. Stunkard, 1984.
20. Jeffery & Wing, 1983.
21. Volkmar, Stunkard, Woolston & Bailey, 1981.
22. Bennett, 1987.
23. Daniels, 1986.
24. Tsujii, Nakai, Fukata & Nakaishi, 1988.
25. Willard, 1991.
26. Bouchard, 1991.
27. Bennett, 1991.
28. Allon, 1973.
29. Blundell, 1990.
30. Garner, Garfinkel & Moldofsky, 1978.

1

**Books, Research and
Popular Diets**

The prime issue in controlling your eating is having a sensible philosophy about eating—not what *techniques* of control to use. We assume that if you are seeking to get better control of your eating you probably already know a great deal about diet and nutrition. People seeking weight control help usually have been on and off diets since their youth. And a large percentage have read dozens of articles and books in the field. Thus, despite the importance of understanding nutritional values, fat content of foods, and eating strategies, reading this sort of information may be redundant and sometimes even damaging. Your compelling desire to be thinner frequently leads to irrational hope for some magic remedy. Many of the books written on weight loss discourage instead of encourage this hope. If you faithfully follow their instructions, you will find yourself eating in ways specifically prohibited by other diet books. If there is any common message found in diet books it is: Eat less of everything (or something) and you will lose weight.

You will find a correct path to eating control after you eliminate the beliefs that make you anxious and depressed. Unfortunately, many weight books give you more irrational beliefs such as the idea that (1) obesity is due to *addic-*

tion to food; (2) obesity results from repressed sex desires, for which you unconsciously substitute food; (3) fatness is an attempt to isolate yourself from love or sex; (4) obesity is a result of a paradoxical attraction to allergic foods (The fat person eats massive amounts of the very foods to which she is allergic); or (5) fatness is simply the result of a bad habit.

Many confusing "remedies" are also suggested—even methods of never being hungry and still losing weight. Supposedly, hunger is nothing more than the result of eating the "wrong" foods, and the simple solution is to consume small amounts of the "right" foods. Unfortunately, few of these simplistic "solutions" to obesity are new—not even in this century. They have obviously not worked, because the number of people with weight problems has increased over the past few decades.

Diet and weight loss books rarely offer anything new. Many of the approximately four hundred weight control books in print in the 1990s apply a single premise or technique to many-sided problems. Many of these books dogmatically state that all people are fat for the same reason; and the same treatment should work for all. Each book offers a "new" principle of diet that is unscientifically tested. The exorbitant claims of most of these books led obesity researchers Jules Hirsch and Theodore Van Itallie to write in *New York* magazine: "We believe it would be desirable if, prior to acceptance for publication, books on diet or nutrition for the public were reviewed for scientific accuracy by several impartial and knowledgeable referees. We find it unfortunate that the public believes that popular diet books contain important nutritional discoveries and that if they are condemned by the scientific establishment it is out of prejudice and jealously."

Early Diets

As noted earlier, the information in most diet books is quite old. The first diet bestseller was called *Letter on*

Corpulence, Addressed to the Public. It prescribed a high-protein, low-fat and low-carbohydrate diet as the solution to obesity. Originally released in 1864, it had sold fifty-eight thousand copies by 1878, quite a bestseller for its time. The first book proposing the low-calorie diet was published in 1916. *Eat Your Way to Health* by Dr. Robert H. Rose, suggesting that calorie counting was the scientific way to lose weight. During the 1920s a diet book was a bestseller for four years: *Diet and Health with Key to Calories*, by Dr. Lulu Hunt Peters. Most subsequent books again and again present a "new" technique or regimen that magically invokes some fat disposal mechanism that we presumably all have. When the authors of these books make any attempt to substantiate their propositions they tend to cite their own success or that of a few individuals. Since this trend seems to be continuing, we recommend a policy of *caveat emptor*: "Let the buyer beware."

Recent Diets

Dietary irrationality is compellingly shown in the estimated seventeen thousand diet methods and plans currently available. Would-be weight losers are besieged by a steady clutter of misleading information and promises. Understandably, people are left feeling betrayed or hopeless. A logical result of illogical thinking! In 1961 Herman Taller had a bestseller with his book, *Calories Don't Count*. His premise was to avoid starches and sugars. This book promoted a diet that was high in proteins and fats and included a cup of polyunsaturated oil a day, which, by itself, amounts to eight hundred calories. Mr. Taller's simple solution was to avoid carbohydrates, a method that was neither new, nor effective, and as we will see, one that is oft replicated.

Dr. Irwin Stillman sold more than 5 million copies of his 1967 book, *The Doctor's Quick Weight Loss Diet.*[1] His procedure was predicated on an assumption that was not based on any scientific evidence, but on his experience with patients he treated. He stated that a diet consisting of virtually all protein consumes an extra three hundred calories a day. While it is true that protein requires more metabolic effort to process, the specifics he presented were unsubstantiated by any research.[2] In addition, his quick weight loss diet failed to address the dangers of a very low calorie, high protein, and high fat diet. There was one notable aspect of his diet program. It was the first modern diet that rejected the orthodox position that there was one right way to lose weight. Unfortunately, the vast popularity of his diet led many people to believe that the Stillman diet was indeed the best way for everyone. Like many dietary fads of the past it offered nothing really new and no real long-term solution. The high fat and relatively low calorie diet was probably effective because of the monotony it produced.

The next major dietary "breakthrough" was presented in 1972. This was the *Dr. Atkins' Diet Revolution*.[3] Dr. Robert Atkins founded his diet on the notion that the "orthodox medical establishment" had conspired to create the impression that calorie reduction is unnecessary. He suggested political activism to stop the medical establishment's overemphasis on calorie restriction, and to begin a new emphasis on carbohydrate restriction. He stated that the dieter can eat as much as he wants, as often as he wants, of rich foods such as heavy cream, butter, mayonnaise, cheeses, and meats. All the dieter need do is restrict his intake of carbohydrates. Despite the fact that carbohydrate abstinence has never been shown, by itself, to be effective for weight reduction, we find it to be a recurrent theme in many diets. However, if one nutrient could be rightly singled out to blame for obesity it would be fats. Animal studies are quite clear on this point. Diets high in fat are many times more likely to produce obesity than are high carbohydrate diets.[4,5] Considering the evidence, the fact that Dr. Atkins's diet is very high in fat makes it quite suspect. If it is effective at all, it is probably a result of individual restraint instead of anything unique to the diet.

One of the first diets that started a new trend in claiming that it served to stimulate the metabolism was *The Doctor's Metabolic Diet* by W. L. Kremer. This was, once again, a low carbohydrate diet, but with a slight twist; it stressed the specific time and order of nutrients. According to this plan one must consume all starches and sugars at lunch. Breakfast was ruled out as useless, and a complete fast was dictated one day a week. Kremer proposed that by periodically changing one's eating cycles, metabolic slowing could be avoided. As with most books of this genre, no scientific or research evidence is supplied to support the author's claims.

Psychologist, Dr. Martin Katahn presents his "answer" to obesity in his book *The Rotation Diet*. He cites as "evidence" for his dietary plan his own seventy-five pound weight loss. This is risky for any health-care professional to do, because we cannot scientifically generalize from a single person's experience. Certainly, it would be unwise for a physician to advocate the use of a new drug simply because it worked on her!

Katahn's diet book does offer some positive psychological strategies however. These include giving up the demand of perfectionism, and avoiding self-downing after a setback. The premise of the diet itself is that if you cycle your caloric intake from very low to slightly high, this will prevent the metabolic slowing (and putting on weight) that can result from your prolonged restriction of calories. The rotation diet, like its predecessor the metabolic diet, makes unsupported claims, but it is the basic low-fat and low-calorie exchange diet.

Dr. Katahn's other very successfully promoted diet was the *T-Factor Diet*.[6] This diet is based on optimizing the body's production of heat; the more heat the body produces the more calories and fat are presumably burned. He suggests that people with weight problems have more body fat because they eat more fat. This contention is not supported by research. However, his view that fat calories efficiently create body fat is accurate. He expands on this truth to propose that calories are not important, but fat intake is. The T-Factor diet, therefore, is a low-fat diet, high in carbohydrates. This diet also takes a rather naive approach to obesity. It tells fat people that they are obese because they have eaten too much fat. An obvious answer is for them to go fatless—which has its dangers.

The Hilton Head Metabolism Diet[7] by Dr. Peter M. Miller is another book that suggests that people can elevate their metabolic rate by following its methods. The author correctly asserts that differences in metabolic velocity is more important in the creation of body fat than is the amount of food eaten. Weight problems are a result of the fact that "fat people do not burn fat as well as thin people." Dr. Miller's answer to this problem of divergent metabolic rates is a low-protein, moderate-fat and high-carbohydrate diet. He also claims that four meals a day and the cycling of caloric levels will rectify slower metabolism. This book, like most diet books, fails to substantiate its specific claims.

Marriage counselor Dr. Bobbe Sommer suggests in her book *Not another diet book: A right brain program for successful weight management*[8] that if you get control of the subconscious forces in the right brain you will lose weight. She says that dieting is not important, overcoming the destructive eating habits that emanate from your subconscious is. Dr. Sommer resurrects the old psychodynamic premise that women unconsciously sabotage their weight to avoid the demands (such as sexual demands) placed on them if they become thin. This diet tends to give all fat people an eating or personality disorder. But research studies widely contradict this idea by showing that most heavy people do not display real eating disorders.

Judith Mazel developed her best-selling plan, *The Beverly Hills Diet*[9] based on personal experience. She "discovered" that one can eat large amounts of delicacies and still lose weight without hunger. She sees hunger resulting from viewing food as comfort and love, a tendency which can supposedly be overcome by bringing together the "cavernous split between mind and body." This book proposes no real solutions that would bridge the "split." Instead, it sets forth a plan by which eating foods in the "proper" order develops "a system of eating based on enzymatic laws."

Like many diet books, *The Beverly Hills Diet* fails to support its claims with any scientific evidence, and Mazel gives no hard data about her "enzymatic laws." She claims that logic is on her side, because in prehistoric times humans could not be particular about the foods they consumed, so no foods could be inherently bad. That is, early humans were too concerned with getting enough of any food, to be selective. Now, following her lead, they can be selective—and presumably thin. But her logic leads her astray, because humans evolved during many periods of deprivation. Survival would be based on the ability to survive on many different types of food taken in any order available. For Ms. Mazel to suggest that the sequence in which food is consumed can inhibit our absorbing it is the same as suggesting that we have an innate dietary defect. Her diet, like others which suggest rearranging rather than reducing one's intake, is not backed by any research data, and doesn't appear to work.

Another diet book that typically ignores current research on eating is *How to Become Naturally Thin by Eating More*[10] by Nurse Jean Antonello. This author makes the assertion that ninety-nine percent of obesity is caused by non-constitutional factors, but gives no proof of this assertion. She claims that because dietary restriction itself causes weight problems, the definitive solution to the dieter's predicament is to eat more. If you stop depriving yourself by eating basic "real" foods as opposed to pleasurable or recreational foods, you will lose weight. As "real" foods that you are welcome to eat any time you want, she lists such high-fat and high-calorie foods as cheese, milk products, nuts, peanut butter, and pasta.

Despite the fact that research shows that deprivation does lead to overeating,[11-13] Ms. Antonello presents a flawed and misleading premise. She promotes the old idea that everyone will lose weight if they just "eat right" and "healthfully." If fat persons simply give up eating for emotional reasons and learn to eat only when hungry, they will become thin. Unfortunately, this is simply not true.

The popularity in the addiction model and the related twelve-step programs has spawned diet books claiming that weight problems represent underlying addictions. Author Kay Sheppard wrote the book *Food Addiction: The Body Knows*.[14] Despite the vast body of research to the contrary Ms. Sheppard asserts that obesity is in fact a symptom of an underlying addiction. The evidence that she offers to support her contention consists of case studies of repeat dieters who binge only to diet and crave food even more. The cases in this book make the obese person sound very much like an alcoholic. In fact, Ms. Sheppard warns the food addict to look for self-denial, compulsions, tolerance, and withdrawal as symptoms of their addiction. As with many in alcoholism treatment, she takes the disease model and proposes that the addiction is a result of a metabolic imbalance—a disease that makes the sufferer powerless in the face of their addiction. Ms. Sheppard inserts some "scientific evidence" to support her claims by suggesting that the illness is caused by consuming too much refined food, which short-circuits the feedback mechanisms in the hypothalamus. Without ever explaining how this happens she moves on to the enkaphelins in the brain and claims that the addiction somehow affects them. She finally inserts information about the well-established connection between carbohydrates, blood insulin and brain serotonin as if this would somehow support the existence of the food addiction. In fact, she provides no evidence of an addiction whatsoever, but she does succeed in labeling all heavy people as disturbed or as addicts.

A remarkably similar scheme was utilized in the best-seller *The Carbohydrate Addict's Diet*.[15] Authors Rachel and Richard Heller offer "the lifelong solution to yo-yo dieting" in their book. These authors in promoting a low-carbohydrate diet offer a strikingly similar model to that offered by Ms. Sheppard to explain the cause of obesity. They suggest that a disorder in the insulin response to carbohydrates results in the carbohydrate cravings after the fat person eats any sweets or starches. That is, in a large percentage of the obese, their bodies release too much insulin when any carbohydrates are consumed. This excess release of insulin into the blood results in a disproportionate drop in blood sugar, which in turn leaves the person craving even more carbohydrates than they first consumed.

One striking flaw in this logic is shown in the case of the insulin-dependent diabetic, whose body produces little or no insulin. Obesity is quite common among people with this disorder. How could this be, if excess insulin were a major cause of obesity? In addition, diabetics who have very high levels of blood sugar have been shown to have intense cravings for sweets. The reason for this is that diabetics (and many obese people) have a cellular insensitivity to insulin. It takes more insulin to force the glucose into the cells. Consequently, sweets and starches may continue to be craved, even though one's blood sugar remains high, because not enough of the blood sugars are getting into the cells.

One is hard pressed to understand how this process, even if it exists the way the authors claim, can be called an addiction. The term addiction refers to a process that begins voluntarily and becomes compelling with prolonged exposure to the addictive substance. What these authors describe is a distortion of the insulin insensitivity that is, indeed, found among many obese individuals. The scientific consensus of this is that it is a concomitant or result of the obesity, but not the cause.

Perhaps the best explanation of the behavior that is

called addiction is found in the book *Breaking the Diet Habit*[16] by Janet Polivy and Peter Herman. These accomplished researchers suggest that dieting itself results in the behaviors commonly attributed to addiction. They provide evidence that all people who practice dietary restraint—both heavy and light—will tend to both obsess about food and occasionally binge. They pose that it is our bodies' active defense of its natural weight, referred to as the setpoint, that results in the frequent loss-gain cycles observed in most dieters. Each time we lose weight our body mobilizes an array of mechanisms to get the lost fat back. Hunger increases, metabolic rate slows, thought of food increases, activity feels less desirable and so on. The authors of many addiction model books suggest that these effects are symptoms of addiction. However, Polivy and Herman demonstrate that slender people who are put on low calorie regimens act exactly the same way as heavy people. So unless we are all addicted to food, few of us are.

The confusion and irrational thinking that tends to be induced by these contradictory treatment guides is illustrated by the following case:

THE CASE OF SAM

Sam began to grow fat at the age of eleven. Until that time he felt he was no different from any other boy. Although he could not recall any trauma event or change in lifestyle that could explain his weight gain, he could distinctly recall that by the beginning of sixth grade he was four feet ten inches tall and 150 pounds. Those measurements were engraved in his memory when he, and the rest of his class, was weighed and measured by the school nurse who told him that he must lose weight. He was not told how or why, but it was made quite clear that something was wrong with him.

His clearest memories of this period in his life was the cruelty of the other children who delighted in calling him fatso, piggy and other names that would reinforce the idea that he was somehow defective. By the end of that year Sam pleaded with his parents to bring him to a doctor to help with his weight. They obliged, and brought him to the family physician who prescribed a stimulant diet pill and handed Sam a standard exchange diet. This was Sam's first exposure to what would be scores of similar diets. The diet pills failed to produce any significant weight loss and Sam had no idea how to implement it, since his mother prepared all the meals, and made no effort to alter them simply because Sam had a diet sheet.

Sam described feeling increasingly desperate throughout his youth as friendships and social activities were punctuated by mocking references to his weight. In the seventh grade he obtained his first diet book: *The Doctor's Quick Weight Loss Diet* by Irwin Stillman. Sam learned that he was fat because he ate too much starch and not enough protein. So for the next two years Sam periodically starved himself on diets of cottage cheese and tuna in water, with an occasional very lean hamburger. He suffered symptoms ranging from extreme fatigue to bad breath from the high protein diet.

After he became discouraged with Stillman's diet, he found another that offered even more dramatic results. By his senior year of high school, Sam had developed quite an expertise in dietetics. In addition to the diet books he owned a dozen calorie and nutrition guides. He was now five foot seven inches and 230 pounds. At this point he read *Dr. Atkins' Diet Revolution*. He discovered that he need not cut back on his fat intake, it was carbohydrates that made him fat. After a year and three attempts at Atkins' regimen he had gained five pounds. He did lose some weight on each of the attempts, but each loss was short-lived. By the time he entered college, Sam grew to dislike himself. He hated being short and fat, and despised his inability to succeed at losing weight.

Sam's next major effort to lose weight came after his first girlfriend broke up with him to date someone else. He was convinced it was due to his weight, so he was ready to try a new diet. He had heard about the exciting results obtained by the liquid protein diets. *The Last Chance Diet* by Robert Linn and Sandra Lee Stuart followed the same logic as Stillman's quick weight loss diet, but took an even stronger position. Pure protein, with no other intake, was the most quick and effective way to lose weight. Sam did quite poorly on this program because the liquid protein made him sick to his stomach. In his depressed state, he began to take a delight in the elation of starvation. All food had become his enemy. His hunger became a marker of success and redemption. In eleven weeks of this he lost sixty-four pounds. Unfortunately, the "last chance diet" had some significant side effects. The liquid protein, which was sold in the form of a pale and mildly sweet viscous solution, lacked several of the essential amino acids. His weight loss involved a great deal of muscle loss. In addition, his skin became dry and brittle, and he suffered from chronic dizziness.

Sam went from 210 pounds to 146, a radical change with radical expectations. Due to his pale and drawn appearance, people would greet him with concerned inquiries such as: "Are you OK?" or more abruptly: "What happened to you?" He began to think this was a result of his not being thin enough. Despite his previously disappointing results he reread Dr. Stillman's *The Doctor's Quick Weight Loss Diet* and decided that it would work this time. It did, and he went down to an emaciated 131 pounds. At this weight his closest friends began assume he was suffering from a progressive and fatal disease. He was hungry all the time and became even more hungry when he ate. The minute amounts of food he would allow himself would result in increased hunger. They were a tease. His sexual interest diminished as he became increasingly obsessed with food. His body was fighting back quite fiercely to bring back the weight that it felt it needed. Over the next eighteen months he gained eighty-two pounds and was once again fat.

Over the next few years Sam would find new hope in the promises of new diets. *Fasting Can Save Your Life* [17] by Ronald Shelton led Sam once again to starve, only to binge all the way back over 220 pounds. *The Immune Power Diet* [18] by Stuart Berger promised that his obesity was a result of an immune system deficiency and could be fixed with a low-fat complex carbohydrate diet. He lost, went down to his "ideal weight," and once again gained his weight back. It was in his last year of law school that Sam read *The Dieter's Dilemma* [19] by William Bennett. He described it as being almost a religious experience. This book, rather than propose another gimmick or short-cut, explained the biology of human obesity. Sam learned from it that his weight was not a result of weakness or character flaw, but of a different biology. He was not inferior but different. He learned that each time he lost great amounts of weight his body began to fight back with such a fury that he would have to dedicate his entire existence to thinness to be able to maintain the loss.

Sam resolved to lose weight once more but this time he picked a basic low-fat, moderate-protein, high-carbohydrate method that he felt comfortable with. He went from 235 pounds to 185. He was still what others might call fat, but he was able to maintain this weight with minimal discomfort. He now accepts himself the way he is, and has not dieted for eight years.

Like many dieters, Sam's irrationality increased as he followed authors of diet books that announce new discoveries that are in no way based on scientific research. Each promising the eager dieter with the new and best method.

We estimate that there have been at least seventy-thousand scientific publications dealing with obesity, eating and weight loss in the past twenty years. To produce diet books which ignore this knowledge is a grave mistake, and unfair to the reader. We will therefore try to integrate some of the salient current research in this field and present it in a way that you, as a non-technical reader can benefit. We shall then focus on how you can change your irrational Beliefs and inappropriate feelings that may stop you from reaching your eating goals. Have you been discouraged by years of false information? If so, read on.

Notes to Chapter 1.

1. Stillman, 1967.
2. Dwyer, 1980.
3. Atkins, 1989.
4. Berry, Hirsch, Most & Thornton, 1986.
5. DuBois, Goodman & Conway, 1989.
6. Katahn, 1989.
7. Miller, 1983.
8. Sommer, 1987.
9. Mazel, 1982.
10. Antonello, 1989.
11. Herman & Polivy, 1984.
12. Herman & Mack, 1975.
13. Wilson, 1991.
14. Sheppard, 1989.
15. Heller, 1991.
16. Polivy & Herman, 1983.
17. Shelton, 1991.
18. Berger, 1985.
19. Bennett & Gurin, 1991.

2

Weight Loss and Health: What is the Relationship?

You may want to reduce your weight to improve your health. This is frequently a good idea, and in many cases leads to a successful outcome. That is, if you do not allow yourself to think of your weight as a disease. That will harm more than help you. If you decide to lose weight for health reasons, watch your inconsistent motivation! Fat people and smokers have much in common in this area. Both are fighting compelling impulses and both are besieged with threats of grave bodily harm if they do not change their ways. Yet these threats often don't work. Interestingly, treatment for nicotine addiction has a far greater success rate than treatment for weight problems. Apparently, improved health is a short-lived motivator for overweight people. Thinking of the benefits of living longer fails to inspire dieters long enough. Better health is often a weak motivator to reduce body weight. As psychologists, we have often found that it is not effective to try to scare our clients into weight loss. The desire to eat and the immediate pleasure of indulging in food seem to offset the later health benefits of weight loss. This is notably true in men, who typically are more accepted when they are physically large than women are, even if their large size is primarily due to obesity. The following case study illustrates this.

THE CASE OF JERRY

Jerry was referred by his physician to one of the authors for treatment for his obesity. He was afflicted with a severe case of sleep apnea, a condition in which he literally stopped breathing hundreds of times a night. A secondary treatment for this illness is weight reduction. Although not caused by being overweight, it is severely exacerbated by it, and weight loss can literally save a life. Even without the sleep apnea, his risk profile was poor. He was just over six feet tall and weighed 380 pounds. In fact, he was told by his physician that unless he lost a significant amount of weight he faced the very real possibility of cardiac failure during sleep. In all respects Jerry appeared to be an intelligent and well-adjusted man. He owned his own business, was married with two teenage children and he reported never suffering from any psychological problems.

During his intake session, he said "I wouldn't mind losing some weight, but it really doesn't bother me." He revealed that he was always a big man and his size seemed natural and appropriate to him. Jerry was prescribed a low-calorie, low-fat diet and weekly rational-emotive group therapy. In his first session he was asked by the group members what he hoped to accomplish in the group. He stated that he would like to lose weight for his health, but other than that, his weight was not a problem for him. Despite his lack of intensity, he initially seemed to be achieving his goal. By the third session he had lost twenty-eight pounds. Although his progress was excellent to this point, the true depth of his low frustration tolerance and irrationality began to show. Jerry owned a small confectionery business and his specialty was premium chocolate. He announced to other members in the group session that he didn't adhere to the regimen because he had to taste the chocolate. He insisted that a single mouthful wouldn't do, he *had* to taste each batch during each phase of the preparation. The therapist and the members of the group encouraged Jerry to resist and find an alternative way to prepare his chocolate. Over the next few sessions, however, Jerry added more to his list of absolutely "necessary" foods to be tasted. He told the group that the only way he could "cleanse his palate" between tasting batches of chocolate was to eat cheesecake. He claimed that its high fat content allowed him to more clearly detect imperfections in the next batch.

Before long, Jerry began to gain weight and claimed that there was nothing more he could do and that the group could not help him as they knew very little about the manufacture of premium chocolate. It was clear that Jerry believed that attendance in the therapy group should have been sufficient effort to promote his health and to treat his sleep apnea. After a couple more sessions in which Jerry politely defended the necessity of his failure to comply with the diet plan, he announced that he would have to leave the group for the holidays. He never returned.

Jerry possessed a number of irrational Beliefs that led to his self-defeating approach to his weight reduction. Some of them were:

"Weight loss is *too hard* if it involves making my job more difficult."

"I *must eat* chocolate, since I am in the food preparation field."

"I can lose weight quickly, so I can always do it *later*."

"I can get away with being overweight and not sabotage my health."

His failure to acknowledge his beliefs and actively challenge them made it too easy for him to give in to the discomfort of self-denial. The act of losing weight involves fighting ones own body and its weight regulatory systems. In order to overcome the powerful force that these systems represent the dieter must be clear about his motives, thoughts, beliefs, and philosophies about weight, eating and dietary restriction. Without this, the dieter will fool himself with irrational Beliefs.

Obesity as a Disease

People are inclined to judge others by their surface image. If your fatness is considered diseased, people will often treat you with contempt. If you and others see fatness as a disease, your being overweight probably leads to lack of self-esteem. Athletes often have a more enlightened view. Like dieters, they also seek to bring about profound physical change. However, they do not begin by defining nonathleteness as a disease.

Fatness is one of the most stigmatized and socially undesirable traits in the western world and is frequently referred to as a disease.[1-3] However, people commonly label any disdained trait a disease. Thomas Szasz compellingly made the point in psychiatry that people with undesirable behaviors are often labeled as having a mental "disease." By adding the stigma of "disease" to the fat person we excuse our own discomfort at disliking them. After all, we don't hate the fat person, we hate his or her "disease."

The great linking of fatness to disease can be traced to the medical profession's attitudes in the 1950s.[4] Medicine decided that obesity was a menace and loudly announced its danger to society. Unfortunately, the victims of this dread disease were confused with its diseased "cause." As we noted earlier, obese people tend to be confused with their condition. They *are* fat. Thus by calling obesity an abhorrent condition, many people see the obese person as abhorrent. In 1951, Dr. James Hundley of National Institutes of Health, stated that "high blood pressure, heart disease, diabetes, and shortened life span are all associated with obesity".[5] Dr. Hundley and other physicians continued making these pronouncements, basing them on the insurance industry data that there is a correlation between weight and longevity. But this still does not show that obesity is a disease. In fact, there have been a number of studies which have documented that obesity is not as harmful as many claim.[6-9]

Indeed, there is a wealth of evidence that fat people suffer an increase in a variety of illnesses. But does this prove fatness to be a disease? After all, African Americans and Native Americans suffer higher rates of heart disease and cancer, yet no reasonable person would imply that being a racial minority is a disease. In a Swedish mortality study[10] it was shown that tall people live longer than short people. To our knowledge few researchers are calling shortness a disease as a result of these data. A more logical interpretation of such a finding is that factors associated with shortness—not the shortness itself—result in decreased life span. There is evidence that obesity and disease operate in a similar fashion. In one study involving more than four thousand people[11] the authors concluded that obesity itself does not explain the increased heart and circulatory disease found among fat people. Instead, there seem to be other risk factors that contribute to the increase in rates of disease found in some obese persons. These factors may consist of sedentary lifestyles, stress levels or dietary insufficiencies, but we cannot conclude that fat itself is lethal. In fact, there are a number of studies[9,12-15] that demonstrate that weight loss does not increase longevity! Ancel Keys, who has studied obesity for nearly forty years, provides evidence that many of the assumed morbidity factors have very little to do with life span. In his study[8] of 11,579 men in seven European studies he found that neither weight, fatness nor physical activity were found to be a significant factor in the 2,288 men who died over the fifteen years of the study.

The results from a population study in Sweden[16] appear to reconcile some of the contradictions seen in the data on obesity and health. This study, which included 1,462 people, found that the type of obesity, rather than the degree, was associated with poor health. As noted earlier, the Body Mass Index (BMI) is a measure of obesity that is based on a height to weight ratio. It is an expression of *overall* fatness, that is not biased by the type or location of the fatness. In comparison, the waist to hip ratio (WHR) gauges a *specific aspect* of fatness, the extent of abdominal obesity. The researchers found that *only* WHR was predictive of illnesses such as diabetes, and respiratory and abdominal infections. Fatness per se was not found to cause disease—but fat in the abdominal area was.

The view that obesity is a disease is further weakened by the fact that many fat people who seem to have been born with a tendency to be obese do not suffer reduced longevity as much as do people who gained weight late in life.[17] Similarly, it was shown that the high rate of obesity found in Polynesians and Samoans[18] is not associated with the increased cardiovascular disease. This research suggests that the relationship between obesity and disease has both environmental and genetic influences.

The doctrine that obesity is a disease leads to the unfortunate trust that many obese persons place in the "cures" offered by the sellers of popular diet books. As suggested earlier, many diet and fat reduction plans are predicated on the idea that body fat is diseased tissue. The fat person is then led to believe that with the proper exercise, potion, food combination, or nutrients, the body will permanently expunge the diseased growth of fat.

Thinness and Health

People who become too thin and those who lose large amounts of weight without satisfactory nutrition commonly suffer health damage. But most people can increase the likelihood of a longer life span by reducing their weight. The evidence suggests, however, that you do not have to achieve an elusive "ideal weight." Popular wisdom states that the rate of weight loss declines as one diets because the "metabolism slows down." This aphorism in fact appears to have a sound foundation. What is interesting is that this metabolic slowing, which is a defense against starvation, is not limited to just weight loss. Rather, it involves every aspect of the life process. Continued weight loss progressively retards life processes. In order to survive a time in which food is in short supply, the body tends to become more efficient and spends fewer calories, thus making weight loss more difficult. Fortunately, if you are continuously under your personal setpoint (your weight when you eat without restricting yourself), this will slow the aging process. Your increased metabolic efficiency slows you down in general, including your disease processes. This occurs irrespective of your starting weight.

A five hundred-pound person losing fifty pounds may actually experience the same proportion of metabolic slowing as a 120-pound person losing twenty pounds. Even though the obese individual is still fat and the thin person is approaching emaciation, both will have lowered blood pressure, less sympathetic nervous inhibition, and slower metabolism. This phenomenon has been documented in adolescent wrestlers who repeatedly lose weight for matches. Those youths who lost for each match had metabolic rates fourteen percent slower than those who maintained constant weights.[19,20] Similarly, formerly obese people have lower metabolic rates than people of the same weights who were never obese.[21-23] Repeated weight cycling seems to enhance this increased metabolic efficiency. With each weight loss and weight regain cycle the body seems less inclined to lose weight and more adept at adding it. [24-29]

Losing weight may be beneficial for most people, but only if done infrequently. In fact, obesity researcher Albert Stunkard stated that one is better off not even trying to lose if they have difficulty maintaining weight loss. [30] His conclusion makes good sense since there is evidence that repeated cycling adds to cardiovascular and related health risks. [15,31,32] Unhappily, many fat people are pressured to lose weight over and over again. This typically results in both psychological and physical harm. Psychologically, it encourages a common irrational belief: "If I repeatedly fail at something as easy and essential as weight loss, I must be a failure as a person." The chronic dieter who keeps regaining lost weight usually begins to rate himself as a global failure as a person. Society tells him that he need only restrain his behavior to be thin, that if he is mentally sound he should be able to control his weight. Yet he fails over and over again. How difficult it is for him *not* to feel like a worm!

Is Dieting Worthwhile?

Dieting may actually sabotage life quality more than obesity does. In a provoking study [23] researchers found that greatly obese individuals who lost large amounts of weight showed signs of starvation, despite the fact that they were still overweight. This and related findings prompted researcher Jules Hirsch to assert that obesity is not a readily treatable condition. [33] His conclusion is corroborated by the work of psychiatrist and researcher Albert Stunkard, who found that no matter how they lose it, virtually all people who lose substantial weight eventually gain it back. This stems partly from the innate or biological factors, but also from the irrational thinking—of both the dieters and the professionals who instruct them. The belief that there is one ideal weight for everyone leads to the setting of unrealistic and unachievable goals. As noted earlier, one doesn't have to reach the "ideal" weight to obtain substantial health benefits. A more moderate goal is sensible for most people. Sadly, if a five foot six inch four hundred-pound woman enters a Nutri-System, Jenny Craig, Weight Watchers or similar diet center she will be told, in all probability, that she must lose more than 260 pounds. This feeds her low frustration tolerance, because she is taught that she must be deprived for years before she really accomplishes her purpose. Fat chance—no pun intended—of her continuing to work for it! The misleading belief that obesity is purely a result of bad eating habits leads to the equally destructive idea that once the bad eating habits are eliminated, so too is your weight problem. How wrong!—as the high rate of fallback among fat people has shown. Consequently, many unfortunate fat people conclude that they have a learning difficulty if they fail to keep their weight down.

Losing weight, particularly if you are quite obese, is often highly desirable. But very overweight people rarely achieve so called standard weights. Why? Because dieting is far more difficult than most non fat people realize. In fact, one author[34] asserts that "human beings, without the most rigid instructions and controls, are not cognitively equipped to monitor caloric intake with anything like the precision required to prevent major changes in body fat stores." In other words, weight loss is so difficult it is beyond the ability of human beings.

When dieters regain lost weight again and again, and when they do not use RET, they usually see themselves as *inadequate people*, when at worst they have *inadequately dieted*. They are really *hurt* when they hear for the first time that they are gaining back weight. They construct despairing thoughts like, "I've gained back weight, I'm weak and no good! There's no way I can stop it! I'm out of control!" These self-depreciating thoughts typically lead to increased eating stemming from what Schacter called the "what the hell effect." The dieter, having globally defined herself as a failure now says "I'm off the diet, what the hell! I might as well keep eating." And she does!

Notes to Chapter 2.

  1. Sobal, 1984.
  2. Wadden & Stunkard, 1987.
  3. Cahnman, 1968.
4,5. Pollack Seid, 1989.
  6. Ernsberger & Haskew, 1987.
  7. Ernsberger & Haskew, 1986.
  8. Keys, Menotti, Karvonen, et al., 1986.
  9. Keys, 1986.
 10. Peck & Vagero, 1989.
 11. Burack, Keller & Higgins, 1985.
 12. Stunkard, 1983.
 13. Garner & Wooley, 1991.
 14. Keys, 1989.
 15. Blackburn & Kanders, 1987.
 16. Lapidos, Bengtsson, Hallstrom & Bjorntorp, 1989.
 17. Van Itallie & Lew, 1990.
 18. Crews, 1988.
 19. Steen, Oppliger & Brownell, 1988.
 20. Melby, Schmidt & Corrigan, 1990.
 21. Stunkard, 1988.
 22. Leibel & Hirsch, 1984.
 23. Leibel & Hirsch, 1985.
 24. Brownell, 1989.
 25. Reed, Contreras, Maggio, Greenwood & Rodin, 1988.
 26. Brownell, Greenwood, Stellar & Shrager, 1986.
 27. Blackburn, Wilson, Kanders, et al., 1989.
 28. Jebb, Goldberg, Coward, Murgatroyd & Prentice, 1991.
 29. Graham, Chang, Lin, Yakubu & Hill, 1990.
 30. Stunkard, & Penick, 1979.
 31. Contreras, King, Rives, Williams & Wattleton, 1991.
 32. Rodin, Radke Sharpe, Rebuffe Scrive & Greenwood, 1990.
 33. Institute for Scientific Information, 1991.
 34. Bennett, 1987.

3

Genes and Free Will: The Psychophysics of Weight

False Premises

The idea that obesity has a significant genetic component is not new.[1] Yet, most approaches treating obesity and weight loss have been based on weak assumptions that seem to ignore this evidence. Myth No. 1: The weight of a fat person results from poor control, while the weight of a slender person results from good self-control of eating. According to this model, the fat person first guides himself by his "real" or physiological hunger. Second, he goes by his habitual or "mouth" hunger. Mouth hunger is regarded as a kind of bad habit that can be unlearned. Should a fat person fail to make herself thin, she is seen as unwilling to make the moderate effort to learn to eat like a thin person, who, by definition, eats the right way—when she is "really" hungry. Another myth is that weight loss is linear and is directly related to reduced intake. A third myth is the notion that maintaining weight loss becomes easier with time.

These myths developed from seeing obesity as quite similar to other behavioral addictions, such as alcoholism, drug addiction, compulsive gambling, and smoking. But obesity doesn't just follow from improper or inefficient behavior. Very simply, eating too much will not make you obese. You will, no doubt, normally gain weight, but within a limited range. This fact was demonstrated many years back by Ancel Keys and his co-workers who experimentally had volunteers overeat and found that few of them became fat. Radical behaviorists believe that if you act undesirably you will change simply by stopping the reinforcements or rewards for your actions. Without reinforcement, your behavior will supposedly extinguish. This approach does not work with obesity for several reasons, the most compelling of which is that the human body dynamically regulates its own weight.

Inheritability of Weight

Some researchers[2-6] have concluded that your body weight is regulated as much by your inherited genes as is your eye color or height. That is, we have little more control over our weight than we do over our skin color. Of course, we can change our weight, but only through a prolonged effort of will and work which our body tends to sabotage! Accepting this premise is important for several reasons. If you acknowledge that your weight is inclined to stay within a limited range whose upper limit usually increases as you grow older, you can prepare yourself to deal with it. However, if you assume that you are fat simply because you have bad eating habits, you may "logically" conclude that if you simply conquer these bad habits you can be thin forever. This is a trap that largely explains dieters' high rate of relapse and regain. If you, instead, prepare yourself for a lifetime—yes, a lifetime!— of conscious weight control, you will be in a far stronger psychological position. If you lose weight and naively expect that all that is necessary for you to remain thin is to occasionally remind yourself of the principles of good eating habits, you would find yourself *gaining* with no effort at all. Your body will do all the "good" work for you!

Some researchers believe that thinness is natural and obesity is an abnormal genetic condition, while others believe that thinness requires a genetically inherited factor,[7] implying that obesity is the natural state. But they largely agree that all of us have a tendency to gravitate towards a biologically set body weight. Virtually every aspect of our metabolism can be shown to be inherited.

Setpoints

The term setpoint was coined by Nisbett[8] who proposed that humans (and other organisms) have biological mechanisms that persistently and vigorously set body weight within close limits. Having a setpoint means, in a practical sense, that the dieter's body will actively resist weight loss, and the overly thin person's body will resist weight gain. When the overweight person loses weight he will then have to fight his body's continuous and permanent efforts to gain it back. Nisbett observed that obese people behave in a very similar way to slender people who are starving. He saw that they frequently attempt to hold their weight beneath their biological dictated setpoint. Like starving people, they have increased hunger, craving for high-fat foods, lower resting metabolic rates, and stronger aversion to exercise. The dieter does not have to relearn "bad" eating habits or to eat "forbidden foods." Her body will take care of that for her.

R.E. Keesey, who has extensively studied the regulation of bodyweight, concluded[9-11] that humans and animals regulate their body weight by employing two basic strategies. The first is changing how we spend our energies. As we gain weight, we tend to be less efficient in the way we burn calories. When we lose weight, the efficiency increases. That is, we expend fewer calories performing the very same activities.

The second way in which we regulate our body weight is through changing our food intake. Research has shown a very large portion of what and how much we eat is regulated by our nerves and body, with free-will or choice as just one other factor.

To understand the concept of the setpoint, imagine a slender sailor who survives a shipwreck and makes his way to a small desert island. After five years on this island, the sailor, who subsists by consuming an occasional fish or coconut declined from his original 140 pounds down to eighty, a new level of thinness with which he has grown to feel comfortable.

Imagine further that after sustaining this eighty-pound weight for several years, the sailor is rescued by a cruise ship. What happens then? Do you think he would stay at eighty pounds or would he rapidly go back to his original weight—or even higher? You are right about the latter guess. This has been the finding of most researchers who have studied this phenomenon. For example, Ancel Keys and his co-workers[12] put conscientious objector volunteers of normal weight on subsistence diets to determine the effects that such diets might have on prisoners of war. The men lost slowly at first but stabilized, even on the subsistence diets. Apparently their metabolic rates adjusted downward to accommodate their prolonged restricted diets. Immediately upon termination of the diet, the subjects moved back to their original weights without making any effort to do so. In this experiment we find that the body actively defends its weight. When through free will, or due to forces outside our control, we are deprived of food, our body invokes mechanisms that work to stave off starvation. We accept this intuitively with thin people, but tend to conclude that this is not the case with fat people. We assume that because we as a society loathe obesity, our bodies do too. Thus, we could come to the fallacious assumption that none of these setpoint processes should come into play with the fat person. But how can our bodies know when we are too fat? Our bodies have never seen the Metropolitan Insurance Company's charts. The three hundred-pound person who loses one hundred pounds, and the 180-pound person who loses the same weight may very well have their bodies react with the same defenses to protect themselves against starvation. And the minute the starvation period is rescinded (or the diet ends) the body uses the same mechanisms to restore its weight.

The tendency of the body to go back to its set weight was confirmed in a series of experiments by Leibel and his co-workers.[13,14] In two studies researchers found that formerly obese people used energy more efficiently than people who had never been obese. People who had always been thin were more physiologically stimulated when they were forced into a state of low blood sugar than would people who were at the same weights who were once obese. Overall, people who were obese earlier in their lives tended to require twenty-five percent fewer calories to maintain their weight than people who had always been thin. In fact, Leibel and Hirsch observed that the physiological responses of obese people who had lost weight were similar to those of thin people who were being underfed. There are some positive aspects of this phenomenon. For example, one study[15] found that runners who were under their setpoint had much higher levels of the beneficial high density lipoproteins than did runners of the same weight who had never been heavy.

This line of research demonstrates some of the ways the human body defends its body weight setpoint. When you lose weight you will require less food, while your craving for food stays the same or even increases. A formerly obese person who eats the same amount as a person of the same weight who was never obese will tend to gain weight. If you were once fat you may actually gain weight if you eat "normally." Leibel[14,16,17] and his co-workers also found that the *location* of body fat affects the setpoint process. They showed that fatness in the hips and buttocks was more resistant to thinning than stomach fat. Our body initiates release of fat from lipocytes by means of our adrenergic system. Fat cells in our buttocks are *more* resistant to messages from this system, which shows that our fat storage and release is not merely regulated by our intake or regulation of calories.

Just as people who force themselves to go lower than their set weights tend to biologically resist and gain again, slender people who forced their weight up have been shown to lose without trying. This was the result of a study with volunteer prisoners by Sims and Horton.[18] They were placed on very high-calorie diets for several weeks. The results showed the falseness of the idea that all people will react to food in similar ways. In fact, some of the prisoners gained considerably more weight than the others. Several prisoners barely gained at all. And all showed a decline in the rate of gaining over time. This demonstrated that people have great differences in how they store body fat. We don't all gain as much or as fast as others when over-eating. Also intriguing is the fact that when people were given access to high-calorie foods, but without the demand that they eat it, virtually all lost weight without trying. What's the moral? As a rule the relationship between eating and weight gain is quite fuzzy. We can state with reasonable certainty that most obese people do not eat as much as most other people assume.

As noted earlier, there is no evidence of a specific style of obese eating. Heavier people do not necessarily eat more food, nor do they choose less desirable foods. This was illustrated by Stunkard and his co-workers, who gave out free coupons to a fast food restaurant to people of all weights. They discovered that obese people did not choose the higher calorie meals more often than the thin subjects.[19] Similarly, Coll and his co-workers performed a study[20] in which people of all weights were observed while eating in several restaurants. The researchers itemized the consumption of 5,000 different foods in nine locations. They found that fat people did not make different food choices than thin people. These findings are contrary to the popular belief that overweight people will tend to choose more fattening food, while slender people will tend to make better food choices.

Some drugs used to alter appetite seem to affect people's setpoints.[21,22] Dexfenfluramine is a medication for the treatment of obesity that has been shown in animal studies to lower their setpoints independent of its appetite suppressing effects. Amphetamines, which have long been used as "diet" pills, also seem to alter the setpoint. This evidence indicates that there is an intimate interplay between our weight and appetite regulatory system, and there is no practical way to separate our setpoint from our eating behavior. However, it is essential to recognize that the collection of weight and fat regulatory processes exist. It lets the dieter understand what he is fighting and how long he will have to fight.

Brain Control

The concept of a setpoint is strongly supported by the research into the neurological control of eating. Damage to specific brain areas, called lesions, can result in huge weight changes. Lesions in the region of the brain called the ventro-medial hypothalamus of mammals will result in an enormous gain in body weight. It will also produce changes in personality, sexual activity and water consumption. When animals are experimentally impaired in this way they become aggressive and violent, and will binge on savory foods. Interestingly, when such animals are given foods with even a slightly "off" taste they act quite finicky. When portions of another brain center, called the lateral hypothalamus, are damaged, dramatic weight loss will ensue. If this occurs in an animal, its behavior becomes strikingly similar to that of a human anorectic. In studies in which rats[23-25] were given lesions in the lateral hypothalamus they became passive, apathetic, and actually avoided food.

The role of the hypothalamus in eating is quite important. Even eating choices that we take to be personal
judgments may actually have their origin in this relatively
primitive brain center. For example, Edmund T. Rolls and
his co-workers observed that cells within the hypothalamus
become active when an animal sees or smells food. These
cells become even more active if the animal is hungry.
Since all of us humans have active hypothalami, it follows
that our conscious perception of hunger, taste, and food
pleasure may very well be based on unconscious neurological functions in this brain center. We can conclude
from this that obese people who chronically restrict their
food intake will often tend to be chronically hungry and
will find food more appealing. They may well have *nerve*
rather than *nervous* reactions!

Social psychologist Stanley Schacter, as well as biological psychologist Anthony Sclafani,[26,27] noted that many
obese humans exhibit behavior that is strikingly similar to
that of rats who have had lesions placed in their ventromedial hypothalamus (VMH). Both the experimental animals and obese humans will eat considerably more than
their lighter weight counterparts when offered highly palatable foods, but will eat less when the foods are tainted.
The VMH rats and obese humans responded more to the
smell and visual properties of foods. Both tended to eat
more when food was easily accessible and eat less when
they had to work to get it. In his article "Some remarkable
findings about obese humans and rats," Schacter notes that
these similarities point to the innateness of behaviors that
may underlie obesity. Changes in the hypothalamus generally result in measurable changes in setpoint that are
independent of changes in eating behavior.[28,29] For example, a person with damage to her ventro medial hypothalamus will gain weight even if eating no more than she
did prior to the injury. When mammals suffer damage in
this brain center their body weight may be permanently
changed.

THE CASE OF GEORGEANNE

Georgeanne was referred to one of the authors for psychological and medical treatment of obesity. Although quite large, Georgeanne presented herself very well at her intake session. She was forty-one years old, five foot three inches and 273 pounds. Despite her size she was dressed quite meticulously, which enhanced her attractive face and hairstyle. With a tone of frustrated sarcasm she told of all the other doctors she had consulted on her weight problem. "I've been on every diet there is, I've even had my jaw wired shut." She went on to describe literally dozens of diets that she had been on since her early teens. These attempts had resulted in nine losses ranging from eighty to more than one hundred pounds, and many more smaller decreases in her weight. Her descriptions of the various diets revealed an extensive and comprehensive knowledge of dietary and nutritional principles. Georgeanne gave an analytical review of every diet doctor and weight loss program she had attended. Although critical of their frequently contradictory and perilous techniques, she never blamed them for her relapses. Instead she professed a belief that there was something wrong with her, a fundamental flaw that resulted in her gradually regaining her weight back after each painful bout of intense dieting.

Each dietary regimen was more difficult and uncomfortable. When the therapist suggested that repeated dieting was encouraging Georgeanne to increase her self-downing, she said, "I like myself, I'm just too fat! I even like my looks, but it's just a major pain in the ass to be this big!" Every aspect of her life was a success. She had a good relationship with her husband, who did not find her weight to be a problem. Georgeanne was close with her daughter, who was also overweight yet happy and doing well professionally. Her recent promotion as a corporate accountant was the last in a series of business accomplishments. In all areas Georgeanne was doing well—except in maintaining her weight losses.

Georgeanne was given the Eating Disorder Inventory, the Minnesota Multiphasic Personality Inventory, the Coopersmith Self-esteem Inventory, and the Zung depression scale. Except for the drive for thinness scale on the EDI, Georgeanne had no psychological problems that could account for her weight problems. In short, she was normal. She joined a RET group and was placed on a seven hundred-calorie-a-day diet. She adhered religiously—as she did on all previous diets—and lost her first fifty pounds in only sixteen weeks. Unfortunately, her rate of weight loss began to slow precipitously. By the fourth month she was only losing a pound per week. In the group sessions she was quite philosophical about her slow losses, and she repeatedly affirmed her resolution to lose at least one hundred pounds and keep it off. Georgeanne was supportive of the other group members, typically exhorting them to stick with the diet program. There was no topic that was too sacred for group discussion, and Georgeanne's openness frequently led other members to disclose and thereby understand the irrationalities that resulted in their emotional difficulties.

Despite her outstanding compliance, Georgeanne lost only an additional twenty pounds over the next four months. She also reported an increasing feeling of malaise—sometimes depression—that had no other source, except for the continual denial inherent in prolonged dieting. At this point Georgeanne requested some individual psychotherapy sessions as an adjunct to the group. During these sessions she shed the optimistic demeanor she set forth for the group, and revealed a saddened and somewhat hope-less outlook. "I don't think I can keep this up, I can't keep starving myself for less than a pound a week." When the therapist suggested that she increase what she was eating so that she would not feel as deprived, she accurately pointed out that if she were losing this little on seven hundred calories, she would probably lose nothing on one thousand or twelve hundred. There was nothing irrational, or demanding about Georgeanne's view. She was working hard, while be-ing subjected to the discomfort of continuous hunger to achieve very little. There was no answer, except a hedonic calculus. That is, how much is getting thinner worth? Georgeanne apparently considered this issue and decided that being thin to please the world was not worth the pain of intense and prolonged dieting. She quit the group and her diet three weeks later. In a subsequent discussion she concluded that the fre-quent attempts to offset her biological predisposition had, with aging, made it nearly impossible for her to lose weight. Not an irrational conclusion!

Although Georgeanne lost large amounts of weight more frequently than most fall-back dieters, her profile is not that unusual. She is an intelligent person, competent in most areas of life, knowledgeable about dieting, yet virtually powerless to maintain a low body weight. What's more, the rate at which she loses weight, despite extreme restriction, is dismal. It is slow enough to make even the most rational person question the utility of abstinence from food. We see in Georgeanne evidence of a biological pre-disposition that is at odds with her weight goals. She loses slowly and gains quickly.

Georgeanne and people with similar histories vainly look for their hidden infirmity, and for a miracle cure. They never find it. The evidence we have presented makes clear that Georgeanne and others like her are fighting their own bodies. They can win, but only if they understand the nature of their foe—the setpoint or the weight regulatory systems. This foe is relentless, tireless, and unforgiving. Conscious effort, on the other hand, can easily be deflected by fatigue, distraction or disturbing emotion. Is such a continued effort worth it? Not always!

Teleology of Obesity

If people who are of normal weight gain back weight losses without conscious effort, why shouldn't fat people? Actually, they should. Fatness may be normal for them. The notion of a biologically set weight does not necessarily mean that there is one correct weight for each height; this is a fiction of life insurance companies. In fact, from a biological point of view it makes much more sense for humans as a species to exist at many different weights. After all, if humans were all slender, famines throughout history would have taken a much greater toll than they did. If everyone were slender prior to a famine, far more people would starve. The presence of people with stored fat may very well represent a genetic hedge against shortages of food.

In addition, it seems that many fat people are endowed with traits that make them more resistant to starvation—which is why these traits have probably always existed. These traits include the tendency to gain and store fat more efficiently, the ability to survive on less food utilizing a more efficient metabolism, and an elevated drive to consume more food when it is available. We can intuitively guess that these characteristics would almost have to exist given the history of humankind. The pursuit of nourishment has been the primary goal of most people across most of our history. To think that characteristics that made some people more resistant to starvation than others would not have evolved is strange. In fact, some authors[30] have likened obese people to "misplaced hunters, programmed for an environment that does not exist in the modern world." They propose that many fat people are suited to survive in a more challenging environment than the one in which they actually live.

The Pima Indians of the American Southwest actually demonstrate many of these principles. Nearly eighty percent of the Pimas are obese and nearly half are diabetic.[31] This high rate of obesity and diabetes are associated with a lower metabolic rate and an insensitivity to insulin.[32-34] This was not the case in the last century. Why, then, did they, as a people, become obese? It seems that with the hardships of forced migration, starvation, and illness those Pimas who were not obese died out. Natural selection does not make aesthetic judgments. If a trait fosters survival, its possessors more frequently survive. In this case obesity was just such a trait.

The view of obesity being adaptive seems to be subtly endorsed by some cultural values. Eastern cultures nearly always depict Buddha as highly rotund. In fact he was quite emaciated as the following quotation makes clear:

> "His limbs became like knotty sticks, his spine which could be grasped from the front through the flabby skin of his abdomen was like the protruding weave of a braid. His protruding thorax was like the ribbed shell of a crab, and his emaciated head was like a gourd that had been plucked too soon."

The distorted depictions of Buddha may be explained by the fact that the cultures that have adopted him as a deity have been exposed to centuries of famines. In these cultures the obese person is revered, and the lean one abhorred.[35] This makes perfect intuitive logic. Attractiveness equals the ability to survive. A person who is less likely to survive the famine, or is too thin to bear a child to term will be seen as less attractive. Similarly, in a society in which fatness represents the ability to provide for one's offspring, a fat man will be more attractive to women.

Notes for Chapter 3.

1. Mayer, 1953.
2. Bennett & Gurin, 1991.
3. Stunkard, 1991.
4. Price, Cadoret, Stunkard & Troughton, 1987.
5. Ness, Laskarzewski & Price, 1991.
6. Institute for Scientific Information, 1991.
7. Costanzo & Schiffman, 1989.
8. Nisbett, 1972.
9. Keesey, 1989.
10. Keesey, 1988.
11. Keesey & Corbett, 1985.
12. Keys, Brozek, Henschel, Mickelson & Taylor, 1950.
13. Leibel, Berry & Hirsch, 1991.
14. Leibel & Hirsch, 1985.
15. Williams, 1990.
16. Leibel & Hirsch, 1987.
17. Presta, Leibel & Hirsch, 1990.
18. Sims & Horton, 1968.
19. Stunkard, Coll, Lundquist & Meyers, 1980.
20. Coll, Meyer & Stunkard, 1979.
21. Stunkard, 1982.
22. Fantino, Faion & Rolland, 1986.
23. Sclafani & Kluge, 1974.
24. Sclafani, 1984.
25. Schacter & Rodin, 1974.
26. Sclafani, 1989.
27. Sclafani & Springer, 1976.
28. Bernardis, McEwen, Kodis & Feldman, 1987.
29. Hallonquist, & Brandes, 1984.
30. Smart & Smart, 1971.
31. Ravussin & Bogardus, 1990.
32. Howard, Bogardus, & Ravussin, et al., 1991.
33. Saad, Knowler, Pettitt, Nelson, Mott & Bennett, 1990.
34. Pettitt, Bennett, Saad, Charles, Nelson & Knowler, 1991
35. Brown, & Konner, 1987.

4

The Fat Personality
Disorder:
Fact or Fiction?

When a person is afflicted with most illnesses, the malady is referred to as a temporary trait. For example, we refer to the state of influenza infection as "having the 'flu'." Similarly, if one develops a malignancy one is said to "have cancer." In contrast, obesity is seen as a disease that becomes an intrinsic and permanent part of the afflicted person.

This becomes strikingly clear when we examine the different names applied to fat people. We do not say that a person has come down with fatness or obesity, we say that he *is* fat, or she *is* obese. This particular use of language seems to be reserved for ailments popularly believed to develop as a result of a defective character.

The open hostility expressed by many individuals towards fat people results from the view that they are different in kind. Fat people are seen as a different category of humanity, not merely people who happen to have more fatty tissue. But there is a hostile paradox within this view. Most people who disdain "fatties" justify their hostility by stating that the fat person has voluntarily gone astray by eating excessively, which is an act of free will. This contradicts the hostility directed at fat people based on their *being* fundamentally different. If people get fat solely

from eating too much, how can we logically conclude that
they are different in *character* in areas unrelated to eating?
In contrast, if they are obese because of their innate characteristics, how can we resent them for having these characteristics! But, perversely, we condemn them, at one and
the same time, for having and for not having free will!

Obesity and Personality

If you are reading this book, it is likely that you have
read other books on weight and eating. As noted in Chapter 1, many of these books take the position that some
defective aspect of the overweight person's psyche is responsible for his elevated weight. Obesity is viewed as a
neurotic symptom, an indicator of an underlying personality disorder.

From the Freudian or psychoanalytic view, you eat
excessively as a result of your sexual energy (called libido)
becoming linked with your oral gratification. You then
have "oral fixation." By this definition, every obese person
is locked into a less mature level of development. Psycho-
analyst Hilde Bruch in her work on eating disorders referred to the fat person as insecure and immature.[1] The
object relation psychoanalysts who suggest that our personality stems from our identifying with significant people
in our early lives, may see obesity as an attempt to feed or
satisfy our mother or father who we have, symbolically,
taken inside.

The behavioral psychologists typically view obesity as
a manifestation of defective reinforcement and learning
(which is how behaviorists explain all emotional disorders).
For example, a behaviorist would infer that an obese person was inappropriately or excessively rewarded with food.
Having learned that enjoying food follows several behaviors, the obese individual will tend to eat more frequently
than a thinner one. We find a similar approach in virtually

all of the schools of psychology which conclude that obesity is symptomatic of some underlying personality problem.

Psychological research presents a quite different picture. Halmi and his co-workers studied a sample of very obese persons who were undergoing gastric bypass surgery —a surgical procedure in which a portion of the small intestine is rendered ineffective, thereby preventing absorption of a large portion of all food consumed. Prior to surgery these patients were given psychological tests to screen them for emotional problems. The results indicated that approximately half suffered from depression to some degree, but less than three percent suffered from any other specific psychological diagnosis. In two similar studies[2,3] subjects were given extensive psychological testing before surgery. The obese people had a few emotional problems, but experienced significant reductions in disturbance following weight loss. As the people who suffered from morbid obesity lost weight, they seemed also to lose their personality disorders.

We can surmise from these results that if people made themselves fat as a *result* of mental or emotional illness, they would be expected to remain disturbed even if they lost weight. After all, how could intestinal bypass surgery make someone less neurotic? Clearly, it cannot. But it seems that the resulting change in body weight did! By becoming thinner these people became more psychologically healthy. This may have been a result of better treatment from those around them, and consequently a change in their beliefs about the world. One thing is clear: these data indicate that emotional problems were not the *cause* of their weight problems.

In another study of people[4] who sought professional help with their weight, twenty-three percent were found to have psychological problems, but seventy-seven percent had none. Perhaps even more significant than the percentages was the fact that there was no difference between the weights of the disturbed and the non-disturbed groups. This suggests that weight is not directly related to the emotional disturbance. This is a common finding in studies of personality disorders and obesity. If fatness resulted from personality or psychological disorders we would expect that the more disturbed one is, the fatter one would get. This has not been shown to be true. Even when massively obese people are given elaborate psychological tests researchers fail to find any consistent personality or emotional illness that would predispose them to obesity.[5] A group[6] of psychologists who studied a large number of people seeking hospital-based treatment for obesity did find that many of the women had scores on a standard psychological test that revealed some personality problem. They found that the obese women were unusually suspicious, socially alienated, and had a tendency to view the world unrealistically. However, these same researchers did not find these propensities in obese men in their study. The fact that they were observed in women, but not men, strongly suggests that the emotional and personality disorders in obese women result from social factors, rather than from obesity itself. Specifically, obese women tend to face far greater levels of social rejection and hostility than obese men. If fat women encounter animosity, condescension, and general poor treatment, it follows that they will tend to view the world in the way the women in this study did.

Although these studies showed some common personality problems, they also found many significant differences. A careful review of the research literature on the personality of the fat person leads us to conclude that there is no unique or specific fat personality. Most of the emotional disturbances that are assumed to cause fatness, seem to *result* from it. In addition, the people sampled in the above studies do not necessarily represent fat people in general. They are people who were sufficiently distressed to seek treatment. When we examine studies of non-clinical populations we observe somewhat different results.

Researchers sampled nearly eight hundred people and found that obese people were *less* anxious than thin ones.[7] This result was repeated in another study by Crisp.[8] Similarly, researchers in Belgium[9] found moderately obese people to be less neurotic, more outgoing, and more non-smoking than slender people.

Rational-emotive therapy (RET) proposes that obesity results from an interplay between a person's biological tendencies and his or her philosophical style. Even if one has a disturbed philosophy, one's fatness is not pathological, because one also usually has a biological disposition for gaining and maintaining extra weight. Without this predisposition the person would be thinner even if she or he had the same disturbing philosophy.

THE CASE OF LAURIE

Laurie had abysmal low frustration tolerance (LFT) that kept her from going through the pain of steadily dieting. But she and her entire family were also at least twenty-five pounds above "normal" statistical weight standards. In other respects, Laurie was a hard worker and rarely damned herself for her shortcomings. So in RET we would call her a person with a somewhat disturbed philosophy and some self-defeating behavior—but not a *seriously neurotic person*. Once she saw what she was thinking and doing, and did *not* put herself down for behaving this way, she was able to use RET to raise her level of frustration tolerance and to do fairly well at dieting.

Intelligence

A common assumption about fat people is that they are less intelligent than thinner people. This belief is held by fat and slender people alike. It is erroneously thought that thin people keep their weight down as a result of superior intellectual control, control which fat people lack. Similarly, the self-downing overweight often endorse this error by thinking that their fatness is inevitable because they lack the character and intellect to reduce it. Soren-son [10-12] published a series of studies examining this matter. His conclusion was that very obese people tend to score slightly lower on IQ tests. However, most of the score differences in the scores can be explained by the social status of obese people. It has long been established that more obese people are found in economically poor groups, and it is also well established that these groups do more poorly on aptitude and IQ tests. Thus, when we adjust for economic differences, we find obese people to have the same intellectual capabilities of slender people. In addition, research makes clear that intelligence is poorly correlated with weight loss. [13] If thinness equalled smartness, then smarter people should lose weight more easily. This is not the case.

The false belief of many obese and self-downing people that they are stupid tends to lead to the additional irrational Belief, "If I try I will certainly fail, so I might as well not even try." The fat person is at a disadvantage for jobs, for admission to school, and for acceptance into social organizations. No wonder this discrimination encourages a wide range of irrational beliefs! Thus, even a gifted and bright person may appear unintelligent if she is socially discriminated against.

Cognitive Style

Belief in External and Internal Control of One's Life

The preceding sections showed that even the fattest bodies are not necessarily created by people's emotional or psychological problems. Obesity is *not* a sign of mental illness. This does not, however, deny that heavy people have *some* emotional differences from slender people. There are several psychological measures of the way people think and view the world around them. These are referred to as cognitive style. Take for example the belief in external or internal control of one's life.

People who have a deep belief in their own ability to change themselves will be more likely to actually try to make a change than those who believe that forces outside their control run their lives.

Smokers tend to think that outside events cause their problems. "Everything gives you cancer." "If your time is up it's up, there is nothing you can do about it." Here the smoker divests himself of responsibility for his own actions, and thereby fails to even make an effort to change his life. A very different perspective is held by the political crusader who marches alone with the protest banner believing that she can change the world. This person probably believes that she has some internal means of controlling things. "If not me who else?" is the essential philosophy of this type of person.

The results of studies trying to find a decisive difference between fat and thin people on a measure of internal control have been inconsistent. Some studies have concluded that there is no difference between the two groups.[14-16] Another study found that if belief in control is broken down into three categories—fatalism, social control, and self-control—obese people did appear to think more externally regarding self-control and social control. But they thought more internally than average-weight people on fatalism.[17] That is, fat people believed more in their ultimate control over their fates.

If there is a difference it might show up in treatment success. Very heavy women believing that external factors control their destiny were found to do more poorly in weight loss treatment than those who believed in the power of internal control.[18,19] Those believing in internal control tended to do better losing weight on their own rather than in formal programs.[20]

One particularly interesting study[21] classified over-weight women as having beliefs in internal or external control. All women took part in a weight-loss program. For the first two weeks, all of the women were given placebo diet pills that would supposedly aid them in losing weight. Later, some of the women were told that the pills were placebos and were encouraged to attribute their weight loss to their own efforts, rather than to the drug. Another group of women were not informed that the pills were placebos and they, naturally, continued to believe that their weight loss success was due to the pills.

The results of the study revealed that women with beliefs in internal control lost weight when they were told the pills were ineffective, but gained weight when they believed that the diet pills were real. The women with external locus of control had *exactly the opposite results*, putting all their confidence in the pills, not in themselves. These findings imply that people who believe they are in control of their own lives tend to give up completely when their control is taken away. Those who believe that their fate is in the control of external forces lose weight more efficiently when they give up personal control.

Overall, the research leads one to conclude that obese people are no different from thin people in their beliefs about control. The typical fat person believes she is just as much in control of her life as the average thin person. But the more strongly a person believes she has ultimate re-sponsibility for what happens in her life, the more likely she is to succeed at a challenging task. So for weight loss the more you have beliefs about internal control, the better you actually control your behavior.

What about you, the person trying to permanently change your body weight. Do you believe your life is in your hands? If you tend to believe that you are a pawn in some cosmic scheme, doesn't that set you up to fail when things start to become difficult? Inevitably there will be times when you are hungry, tired, and frustrated. Add to these feelings the underlying belief that change is not under your control and you will be much less inclined to work for it. On the other hand, if you fundamentally believe in your ability to overcome obstacles, then you will more readily try to overcome adversity.

THE CASE OF ANN MARIE

Ann Marie believed that her important goals, especially her sticking to a healthy low fat, low salt diet, were not in her control, because she had failed to adhere to such a diet on numerous occasions. She thought that she was *unable* to stick to her diet because her strong tastes for fatty, high salt food overpowered her and *made* her go back to eating them. She also thought that very bad Activating Events (A's) in her work life and her love life *made* her too weak to withstand her hunger pains and *drove* her back to improper eating. When Ann Marie went to a Rational Recovery group she learned that *she*, and not her taste buds or her bad experiences in love and at work, drove her to poor eating habits. Once she put *herself* in control, she was able, with no anguish, to give up fatty and salty foods and only occasionally fell back.

Internality, Externality and Restrained Eating

In 1968 social psychologist Dr. Stanley Schacter proposed that a fundamental cognitive difference between obese people and slender people is the way they respond to external stimuli. According to his theory, externally oriented people will be more likely to decide to eat based on events taking place outside their body. Thus, the sight, smell and taste of food will be far more provocative to the fat person than to the average weight person. A highly external person may entirely forget to eat unless he receives cues from things around him. Such cues may be the clock indicating that it is "lunch time," seeing other people eating, the scent of cooking food, or taking a small taste of something, only to find you are hungry for more.

In a classic study by Albert Stunkard[22] obese and average weight people were asked to swallow balloons that were hooked up to a pressure monitor. All subjects were asked to report if they were hungry every fifteen minutes. The results indicated that average weight people were more likely to report hunger when they had stomach contractions than heavier people. This suggested that heavy people were less attuned to their own internal hunger signals, and more synchronized with external cues. Supporting his findings was a study in which heavy people were observed in a restaurant serving food buffet style.[23] The amount that they would eat would change based on whether they were alone or with company, and also on how much their companions ate. They would eat more when alone or in a familiar place. In a related vein, researchers found that fat restaurant patrons[24] tended to order a particular dessert in a restaurant when the waitress provided an appetizing description of the dessert and encouraged the diner to order it. Nonoverweight customers were much less affected by the waitress's recommendations. Girls in a summer camp were found by researchers to have a link between externality and weight. The researchers measured their sensitivity to external events using memory, emotion and food cue tests. The results indicated that the girls who were the most sensitive to external environmental events tended to gain the most weight in the camp.[25]

Many other researchers have found evidence to support Schachter's proposed link between externality and obesity,[23,24,26-28] even in children as young as seven years.[29] Yet, some contest the connection between fatness and externality, and come to a somewhat different conclusion with the same evidence. These researchers suggest the external sensitivity[29] is a result of the act of dieting itself. People who routinely restrict their eating—whether or not they lose weight—tend to be more concerned with food. This concern is believed to result in a hypersensitivity to food cues.[30] The fact that slender people who chronically diet exhibit the same external behavior as do fat people provides powerful evidence for this position.[31,32] Thus, another disagreeable trait attributed to fat people may have nothing at all to do with being fat, but very much to do with the intense pressure placed on fat people to be different.

The pressure to be thin leads to the chronic and prolonged restraint of eating, and ultimately behavioral and psychological change. Restrained eating has been shown to be a major cause of bingeing[33] and other apparent pathologies in eating behavior. By restraining eating, for weight loss or for other reasons, the individual increases hunger. The maintenance of this hunger takes cognitive and emotional effort that eventually results in a fatiguing effect. When this occurs a release of the restraint tends to lead to an overcompensation. We see this in virtually every animal that has been deprived of food; when allowed to eat it will binge. Polivy and Herman demonstrated one way this occurs in dieters.[34] Dieters (restrained eaters) and non-dieters were given either one or two milkshakes prior to tasting ice-cream, while some were given nothing prior to the tasting. They were told that the milkshake consumption was part of a taste perception experiment. The results were surprising. The dieters who had no milkshake ate less ice-cream than the non-dieters. While the dieters who had one milkshake ate more ice-cream than the non-dieters, and those that had two milkshakes had even more. Thus, when the dieters felt that they had gone off their diets by having a milkshake, they tended to give up control when tasting the ice-cream. After having two milkshakes (which should have left them reasonably full) they ate nearly twice as much ice-cream as did the dieters who did not have any milkshakes. Thus, when we believe we have failed at restraint we tend to say "WHAT THE HELL" and eat until we reach binge proportions.

No Real Differences

Overall, the research indicates that the main difference between overweight people and slender people is that the overweight people are fatter. The irrational behaviors and emotional problems that we may observe in fat people appear to be a result of being fat in a society that disdains fat and those that wear it. The next chapter will elaborate on this premise

Notes to Chapter 4.

1. Bruch, 1981.
2. Chandarana, Conlon, Holliday, Deslippe & Field, 1990.
3. Larsen & Torgersen, 1989.
4. Fitzgibbon & Kirschenbaum, 1990.
5. Webb, Morey, Castelnuovo Tedesco & Scott Jr., 1990.
6. Johnson, Swenson & Gastineau, 1976.
7. Hallstrom & Noppa, 1981.
8. Crisp & McGuiness, 1976.
9. Kittel, Rustin, Dramaix, DeBacker & Kornitzer, 1978.
10. Sonne, Sorensen, Jensen & Schnohr, 1989.
11. Sorensen, Sonne, Christensen & Kreiner, 1982.
12. Sorensen & Sonne, 1985.
13. Kincey, 1983.
14. Mills, 1991.
15. Davis, Wheeler & Willy, 1987.
16. Nir & Neumann, 1991.
17. Thomason, 1983.
18. Weinberg, 1984.
19. Rabkin, 1982.
20. Hankins & Hopkins, 1978.
21. Chambliss & Murray, 1979.
22. Stunkard, 1976.
23. Maykovich, 1978.

24. Herman, Olmsted & Polivy, 1983.
25. Rodin & Slochower, 1976.
26. Kozlowski & Schachter, 1975.
27. Rodin, 1981.
28. Widhalm, Zwiauer & Eckharter, 1990.
29. Costanzo & Woody, 1979.
30. Polivy, Herman & Warsh, 1978.
31. Herman & Mack, 1975.
32. Herman, 1978.
33. Williams, Spencer & Edelmann, 1987.
34. Herman & Polivy, 1984.

5

Society's Views of Fat People: Prejudices and Discrimination.

We judge a book by its cover, and often ascribe personality characteristics to people according to their various shapes and sizes. That is why your weight is important above and beyond romantic and sexual relationships, and why it affects your educational and occupational success. After all, if fatness were only viewed as the outward sign of some people's efficient metabolism—which it largely is— we would draw few conclusions about fat persons' character or talents. We might still choose our lovers according to their size and beauty, but our choice of friends and co-workers would not similarly be influenced.

Exactly what traits and attributes fat represents has drastically changed throughout the ages, which suggests that the relationship between weight and personality is "found" in social definitions rather than in facts and is not firm. However, various relationships have always been dreamed up.

Since the time of cave men and women, and up to the industrial revolution, humanity has been in constant pursuit of food. Dieting was not an issue, primarily because there was not enough food around for obesity to become a problem. Food shortages and periods of famine were accepted facts of life. Many dreamed of having all the food they would want to eat and enjoy, and losing their gaunt looks in favor of prosperous plumpness. Heavier persons were admired and envied; they were obviously able to procure larger amounts of food than others, perhaps with less physical exertion, perhaps by benefiting from others' labors. Weighing more than others was seen as having positive characteristics, such as wealth, wisdom, or strength. As recently as the 1850s, "abundant flesh symbolized all that was best in middle class life, especially its comfortable prosperity . . . Plumpness symbolized a clean, temperate life."[1]

We have come a long way, at least in western society, from having to struggle to obtain food. We have reached a level of economical growth where some of the poorest of us can afford to, and often do develop fleshy bodies. But as it is no accomplishment in today's world to acquire a great deal of food, we have shifted our aesthetic preferences from valuing plumpness to pursuing thinness. Being slender has become a symbol of strength and self-control (self-denial), the ability to resist the culinary temptations surrounding us.

Before the industrial revolution hard work was unavoidable for most people, necessary for survival, but not necessarily admirable. It was more admirable to be rich and inactive and to be able to enjoy life at a leisurely pace. But now that we no longer have to engage in hard physical labor for our daily living, we have come to value work and achievement. Those who work hard, even though they could get by without doing so, demonstrate a "superior" drive or life force. We admire hard-working go-getter people, who make their own millions, rather than those who have inherited money and do not accomplish much on their own. Being active, goal-oriented, in control of ourselves as well as of every situation, are now considered desirable traits. A thin, well-toned body supposedly presents the image of a person in control of his or her destiny.

Studies find that thinness has become a symbol of

competence, intelligence,[2,3] assertiveness, higher socio-economic status,[4] and self-control.[4,5] Conversely, fat is seen as a sign of gluttony, self- indulgence, weakness of character, and even antisocial behavior. Overweight people are thought to be an "emotional mess," eating to assuage their feelings of inferiority, insecurity, and sexual inadequacy.[6] In one study for example, college students viewing pictures of normal weight and overweight males and females judged that the overweight persons were less attractive, less likely to be dating, lower in self-esteem, more emotional, and deserving of a fatter, uglier partner than normal-weight persons.[7] Studies find that non-fat people attribute to obese persons negative personality characteristics even if they know nothing about them.[8,9] Women, adolescent girls, and the morbidly obese are particularly likely to be the target of such negative judgments.[10,11] Subjects asked to write stories about overweight characters tend to write sad or negative stories and to endow the characters with unpleasant personalities, especially when the overweight character is said to be a female.[12]

Prejudices and Stereotypes

The strong prejudice that exists against obese persons is evident for children as young as six years of age.[11] In studies of reactions to various handicaps, adults and children were presented with simple black and white drawings of the following: a "normal" looking child, a child with a brace on one leg and leaning on crutches, a child sitting in a wheelchair with his legs covered by a blanket, a child with a hand missing, a child with facial disfigurement on one side of the mouth, and an obese child. In repeated studies, using boys and girls, men and women of different ages and socio-economic backgrounds, living in cities or in rural areas, handicapped or not, the overweight child was considered least attractive, and, perhaps more importantly, least likeable.[13-15] Unlike the children with the various physical disabilities, the fat child was seen as responsible for his appearance, and a whole set of undesirable personality traits were attributed to him. Subjects in these studies saw themselves as being most dissimilar from the fat child.

Society disapproves of fat, and tends to blame fat people for their condition,[16] unless they can demonstrate an "excuse" for their weight, such as a glandular disorder.[17] Fat people are viewed as sinners, criminals, ugly, disease-ridden, and mentally unbalanced.[6] Fat is a sin because fat people are "bad" people—gluttonous and self-indulgent. Self-restraint and self-denial have always been important in American life. In the modern version of morality, however, gluttony often appears to be even more sinful than sexual immorality. If a friend calls you up and confesses that she was "very bad" last weekend, the chances are that she is referring to going off her diet in favor of some "sinfully delicious" deserts. There is also the popular view that heavy women are more sexual, so that their weight is a sign not only of oral, but of sexual gluttony as well. Historians tell us that in the early 1800s fragility and slenderness denoted purity in women, and indicated "higher passions" of a spiritual nature in men.[1]

Interestingly, the opposite view has also recently been held. While plumpness in the 1950s was a sign of clean living, thinness was identified with romantic excess, degeneracy and lack of control over one's "animal" passions. The *femme fatale's* slenderness reflected her evil, dangerous nature. Rather than being ethereal, thinness was considered Satanic.[1]

Just as in the 1950s skinny people were viewed with suspicion, we now have become unaccepting of fat persons. Because we decide that we do not like fat, we go on to conclude that those who dare be fat, dare go against our standards, are antisocial, almost criminal.

"It isn't a crime in America to get fat—but it might as well be . . . You can steal a million dollars or beat your wife in private and still be socially acceptable. Let yourself get fat in public, however, and you will find the finger of scorn continually pointing at you or punching you in the tummy. It is hard to figure why, when a man gains weight, his friends should take it as a personal insult to them, but that's the way it is."[6]

THE CASE OF HAL

Hal didn't mind doing poorly at his teaching job or failing to get his Ph.D. degree after he had worked— and not worked—at getting it for almost ten years. But he went to the gym four times a week and did a great deal of boxing. He weighed almost two hundred pounds—all muscle. If he gained a pound or two of fat, his peers at the gym would tease him mercilessly about this. Hal almost went berserk at these times, hated himself immensely, and punished himself severely and deliberately by eating rotten food and staying away from the gym and from boxing. This, of course, tended to make him gain more weight.

Hal, in the course of twelve RET sessions, was shown how prejudiced the world—and *he*—was against fatness, and how he could set reasonable weight standards for himself even if some of his athletic friends were still horrified when he gained some flab. By changing his impossible ideals, and by learning to fully accept himself with some fatness, Hal was able, for the first time in his life, to live a largely unanguished life.

Because obesity is so highly visible, fat people are greatly reviled. Perhaps because obesity is "out in the open," people feel that they can express their views about fatness openly as well. Extreme negative feelings against fat persons are voiced clearly and unabashedly. For example, one of the authors observed T-shirts being worn in New York City recommending that we "Save the whales,

harpoon fat chicks!" According to these sentiments, the sin
of overeating, or more likely just having an overly efficient
metabolism, is almost punishable by death.

Fat people, it is commonly held, should be punished
because they offend our aesthetic sensibilities. They take
up too much space on subways, buses, airplanes, and
elevators. They consume more than they contribute to
society. They become ill and need to be taken care of, or
they die early and their families are left unsupported.[6] The
only way fat people can gain some acceptance and forgive-
ness for their crime of overeating is to at least try, or look
like they are trying, to lose weight. They must never eat an
ice cream cone in public, never be seen eating a normal
size portion of non-diet food!

Does being overweight really make one less than
human? When we are thin, are fat people simply easy
targets for venting our frustrations, for making us feel
better, in comparison, about ourselves? It is very human to
want to feel "better" or "superior" to others. Rather than
accepting ourselves with our talents and flaws, many of us
think we must be better than others in order to lead a
happy existence. Especially when feeling down or insecure, we may look for someone to compare with favorably.
At the same time, we may feel guilty about putting others
down, and we may quickly dispose of this guilt by blaming
heavy (or otherwise disadvantaged) people for their predicament: "Yes, they are worse off than I am, and it is their
fault. It is their fault that they are fat, and they deserve my
disdain."

Everyone feels entitled to comment about others'
weight. Relatives and friends, in the guise of "good will,"
make a point of noticing any weight gain, and telling you
"for your own good" to stop eating like there's no tomorrow. Perhaps it is partially good will, though such comments are rarely helpful, neither for the heavy person's
ability to diet, nor for his self-concept. Perhaps it also
makes these relatives and friends feel self-righteous, per-

haps they can (erroneously) feel superior at least in this one area. It is of course no accomplishment to be thin when your body naturally tends to achieve that state. A normal weight person can be proud about keeping those ten pounds away that always try to creep back on the scale, but she cannot legitimately compare herself to someone who has had a weight problem since childhood, and would have to be in a constant state of starvation to reach "normal" weight.

Why People Create Prejudices and Stereotypes

Since being fat is now considered a negative trait, we could feel empathy for fat persons, encourage them to lose weight, and teach them to like themselves even if they do not do so. To some extent we do this, but we also wonder how come some people turn out to be fat, and how come some people are handicapped or have other problems. And we worry about *ourselves*. What if it happened to *us*? Indeed, if misfortunes occur randomly, they could easily happen to us. Because it is threatening to think that bad things could happen, we invent a "belief in a just world":[18] fat people or handicapped people must have something very wrong with them, or must have done something very wrong, and they therefore *deserve* their fate.

We make global judgments about people's worth based on their fatness or their handicap (rather than believing that they are regular people with extra fat tissue or with a handicap). We then give the fat or handicapped person responsibility for his predicament, and we can feel that this would never happen to us, since we are good people, favored by the gods. The belief in a just world gives us a false sense of security. As long as we act reasonably well, no great misfortune will befall us. Since it is not a realistic belief, however, when an unforeseen tragedy does befall us, we will blame ourselves for not being worthy of a better fate. Also, when we unfairly blame others for difficulties

they largely do not control, we create poor social relationships.

Humans tend to be ethnocentric—to see positive
characteristics in people in their own ethnic or religious
group and to see negative ones in members of different
groups. This is a form of narcissism, the belief that those
similar to us are better than those who are different. But it
is also a self-protective mechanism, to guard against people
who are different and may act badly to us. Just as we give
negative traits to people with different features and skin
color, we also do so to people who look different because
they weigh more. They are different, therefore they are
undesirable. Not only do we decide that the trait of fatness
is undesirable, but we attribute a whole host of other
negative characteristics to heavy persons, and label them
as overall undesirable *persons*.

Humans also think differently about their own behaviors and characteristics than about others', because we
really can't *see* other people's inner motivations and
choices. We see ourselves making certain choices when we
react to outside events, but we don't know what goes on in
others' heads. So when we see that they are acting in
certain ways we wouldn't choose ourselves or when we see
them looking different from us, we wrongly conclude that
they are different *inside*. Thin people erroneously think
that fat people have many personality characteristics that
are different from them, aside from the difference in
weight. Their extra weight, it is thought, *must* have come
about because of their different, less desirable personalities.

Discrimination

As a result of the prejudices against fatness, there is
much discrimination against obese persons in both academic and work settings.[6,11] Research has found that obese
high school students are less likely to be accepted into

college [19,20] even though their academic qualifications are the same. Even when they believe that an overweight person is equally well qualified with a thinner one, employers are more likely to hire the thinner applicant.[21] One study which measured attitudes towards hiring obese women [22] found that sixteen percent of employers surveyed would not hire obese women under any condition, and another forty-four percent would not hire them under certain circumstances.

Another way of measuring possible discrimination is to compare the salaries of thin and fat persons, all other things being equal. One study [23] found in its sample that only nine percent of executives earning $25,000 to $50,000 were ten pounds or more overweight, while thirty-nine percent of those making $10,000 to $20,000 were similarly overweight.

Many obese persons have testified to such discrimination.[24] The true extent of weight related discrimination cannot be measured because employers are not likely to admit to their own biases.[6,23]

In one clever study,[25] pictures of female college juniors, accompanied by a description of the student's interests and scholastic achievements, were sent to a group of employed men, who were asked to estimate the chances of that student being accepted to graduate school. Some of the pictures depicted overweight students, others were of normal weight females. Not only were the men less optimistic about the chances of the overweight women's going to graduate school, but they were also less likely to bother to complete the survey when the target picture was of a heavy student. The men in this study responded with their own prejudices, and perhaps also considering the prejudice that they expected the overweight students would encounter from the graduate school admission board.

Research finds that people's prejudices influence their ratings of obese salespeople, and diminish their desire to work with obese salespeople, especially with obese

saleswomen.[26] In one study students were asked to take
the roles of being regional sales managers and were asked
to place recruits in one of three territories. Two of the
territories were high-volume placements, while the other
was a rural area with few good accounts. A sales recruit
described as extremely overweight, particularly a woman,
was more likely to be assigned to an undesirable territory
or not selected at all, regardless of her other accomplishments or talents.[27]

In another study, college students viewed videotapes
of overweight and normal weight men and women performing various tasks in arithmetic and mirror drawing,
and rated them as job applicants. Overweight applicants
were less highly recommended despite identical performances. These prejudiced recommendations derived from
the rater's judgments of fat people's personalities or from
their concern that an overweight employee would look bad
to others.[28]

Of course images are often deceptive. Many thin
persons are not successful or accomplished and many fat
persons are, but still we make generalized judgments
about fat people's character or lack thereof. This leads to a
kind of self-fulfilling prophecy; fat people may indeed become less accomplished, because they get fewer opportunities to show their talents. Here is a case study of a fat
person who faced a great deal of discrimination, but in the
end was able to find a workplace where her talents were
acknowledged.

THE CASE OF JANICE

When Janice first consulted one of the authors she
was in her mid-thirties, attractive, highly articulate
and just under 300 pounds. Her height, which was
well above average, gave her an appearance of being
very large rather than obese. And after talking to her
for a short while it was clear that she was a capable

individual. In addition to having an advanced degree in a health related field, she was an honors graduate from a major university. Her work as the highest official in a charitable organization had won her praise and acclamation as a major figure in her field. She said she was pleased that she had reached the point that people now knew her as Janice, not a fat lady. But this had not always been the case.

Her professional history was marred by repeated setbacks as a direct result of her weight. Each time was more painful than the previous. What made it especially difficult to deal with is that unlike racial or religious prejudice, the bias against her weight was more open and more direct. After all, it is not illegal to discriminate against fat people. Her first job after college was in a job counseling agency. In such a field the highest paying jobs were those that involved meeting with the corporations who would hire people her company would represent. Her position as a counselor entailed primarily telephone work. After a year and a half getting excellent reviews from both her superiors, co-workers, and clients, she asked for an opportunity to work as the higher level corporate representative. Her boss avoided the subject for a while, until finally she pressed the issue. His response was something to the effect that she didn't present the right image. She knew what he meant: she was too fat to represent the company.

That painful rejection was the impetus for Janice to go ahead with graduate school in social work, something that she had wanted to do for a while. She graduated with honors and took a job with a religious charity. Janice shared an office with Ann, a very attractive woman who was of a different faith than that of the majority of the woman. In fact Ann looked very much like the ideal WASP fashion model.

This became quite significant when both ended

up competing for the position of regional associate
director, a highly visible job that required meetings
with donor organizations. Janice was certain she
would get the job; after all she had received better
evaluations, produced more reports and instituted
more innovations than any other person who held her
same job. Ann was given the promotion. Shocked and
dismayed she went to the director of the charity who
very euphemistically told the same thing as her last
boss did: An elegant variation of "You are too fat!"

Janice did become thinner, she lost 50-60
pounds a couple of times but realized, after much
suffering, that the effort of losing weight took energies
that she could more profitably direct elsewhere. At
last contact Janice headed her own charitable foundation.

Self-Imposed Consequences of Discrimination

Fat people often come to feel that they *deserve* to be
discriminated against. They are not necessarily more enlightened about the causes of their obesity than the rest of
society. However, they do know that they are not good at
losing weight, not good at keeping it off. They conclude
that there is indeed something wrong with them. They are
not "as good" as other people. Obese adolescent girls, for
example, feel and act as members of racial and ethnic
minorities often do, exhibiting withdrawal, passivity, the
expectation of rejection, and over-concern with their self-
image.[6]

Fat people try to hide their fat, because they don't
want to suffer the real—and sometimes imagined—rejection and contempt of others. They feel embarrassed about
exercising in public, revealing their bodies in skimpy gear,
and perhaps letting people know that they get easily tired.
But how to get in shape without exercising?

Many fat people, as well, try to hide their bodies in

every day life. They feel little incentive to dress fashionably and show off their large bodies, though clothing is a
means of communicating about one's tastes and personality. A large body can make a bold fashion statement, but
showing it off requires that the fat person is comfortable
with the label "fat." It requires acknowledging that some
people may be disapproving, but nevertheless accepting
and approving of oneself. Instead, fat people often hide in
nondescript clothing, hoping to go unnoticed. This often
brings on less acceptance of fatness by prejudiced ob-
servers.

How comfortable is a three hundred-pound woman
likely to feel eating in a restaurant? Would she only be
imagining that her measurements are being taken by curious neighbors, that the caloric content of the food she is
eating is being counted, and the speed with which she
ingests is being evaluated? Chances are, some of this is
going on. Most fat persons dread eating in public. They
fear the curious stares, the negative evaluations. Of course
they could choose to ignore these, but that would require
very strong resolve and rational thinking.

The National Association for the Advancement of Fat
Acceptance (NAAFA) has members who are mostly quite
overweight. This group has monthly meetings over dinner,
but special rooms are reserved for this purpose. The lead-
ers of the organization know that many members would
not eat in public alongside normal weight people. They
would feel unable to handle the stares, and they would feel
obligated to have only the lightest of fares, to prove that
though they have committed the horrible crime of becoming fat, they are at least now repenting and attempting to
reduce.

A president of NAAFA told the authors of times when
comments were made behind her back about her weight.
She would usually ignore these comments, but sometimes
she would confront the whisperers. One thin woman in a
restaurant whispered to her spouse, "Look at how fat she

is!" The overweight president of NAAFA turned to the woman, stood very closely, and said, "Yes, I am very fat!" She was implying that though she was fat and, indeed, she herself would have preferred to be thinner, she had a right to be fat, a right to lead a life without others gratuitously damning her.

Fat people require a great deal of emotional strength to be able to confront those who make negative comments or allusions about their appearance; and they must have unusual self-acceptance to ignore bad mouthing without making themselves enraged and self-loathing. Knowing that they face a great deal of hostility and little friendliness in the world, many fat persons become recluses with very limited lives, never to develop themselves professionally or socially as they would in a more accepting world. Later in this book we will discuss ways of handling this difficult situation and making the best of it.

Fat people also require great emotional strength and wisdom to patiently override negative first impressions, and allow closed-minded people to overcome their own limitations, and then see the full person behind the fat, with as much to offer as anyone else. As noted above, people are prejudiced because they fear anything different, especially something they see as negative for themselves. However, prejudices can be overcome with time. The greatest harm occurs when fat people internalize others' negative views of fatness and give up trying to change their agreeing with these views. They may believe the fallacy that there is power in numbers: "If many people have negative things to say about me, I must be somehow inferior. They must be right."

While very overweight persons are stared at in restaurants, slightly chubby people are probably not given much attention. However, being that so many people unreasonably *think* that they are overweight, many chubby individuals make themselves self-conscious of eating, or even of just being in public. They feel ashamed of not being thin, and the drive to cover up their shame overshadows their desire to live an active life. Plump or fat people often make the same generalization as do those who see them from the outside: "Because my fat is undesirable, I as a person am undesirable. Being undesirable, why even try to do much of anything?" It would take great creativity to "logically" explain how a person's weight equals a person's worth (i.e., the thinner, the more worthwhile), quite aside from a host of other traits and characteristics she or he possesses. However, many heavy persons have a gut feeling, albeit unexamined, that they *are* their heavy weight. In later chapters we discuss how you can rid yourself of such self-defeating and irrational views. At this point, we note that discrimination against yourself can come from inside as well as from others.

Hal, whose case we examined earlier in this chapter, was only looked down upon by his athletic friends when he gained a few pounds of flabby weight. All his regular friends, male and female, thought he had a great build and looked at his muscles rather than his flabbiness. But he, his own worst enemy, downed himself severely before he learned RET, for even the slightest increase in his flabbiness.

Who Stereotypes Most

Not everyone is equally prejudiced against fatness, of course. One study found that persons with anti-fat attitudes tend to be more authoritarian, politically conservative, racist, in favor of capital punishment, less supportive of nontraditional marriages, and less tolerant of sexuality among handicapped, homosexual, and elderly persons.[29] Perhaps we can say that prejudiced persons "think small." They are more rigid, more convinced that there is only one right way to run a country, one proper way to live one's personal life, and only one acceptable way to appear. Once they have concluded that fat is "bad" because it deviates from the norm, prejudiced people attribute many moral flaws and disturbances to fat persons, and encourage their being condemned.

One way to overcome stereotypes is through exposure. Getting to know people from another culture or race allows us to see that though there are certain differences, there are unique individuals within each culture, and few fit the preconceived stereotype. Similarly, people who for one reason or another have known several obese persons learn that they are different from each other, that they are just as complex as the rest of us, and that any simple generalization does not come close to describing them.

Knowledge of the complex nature of obesity also helps dispel some of the negative views of heavy persons, the sense that they are guilty for overeating, or that their weight is a reflection of warped psychic make-ups. Thus adults are less likely to blame fat persons for their predicament than children are.[30] In particular, adults who have taken the trouble to learn about the true causes of obesity are less blaming. However, persons with misconceptions and anti-fat attitudes can be found everywhere. Even mental health practitioners (particularly if they are female, younger, and not overweight themselves) are more likely to assign negative psychological symptoms to their obese clients than to normal weight clients.[31]

Truth Behind Stereotypes

Though there is such a strong consensus about fat people having different, less desirable personalities, or having more psychopathology, research has failed to find much of it. Overweight persons in the general population show no greater psychological disturbance than do non-obese persons.[10,11] Theories about emotional factors leading to obesity were developed by clinicians who had their own biases. As in all areas of science, individuals develop theories based on their own experience, and their own unique interpretation of the information they perceive. But science also involves testing these theories. Often theories are wrong, and usually they are disproved and discarded. However, in the case of unraveling the causes of obesity, clinicians seem to have ignored the facts, the facts being that there is little relationship between obesity and psychopathology. It is true that if fat persons do experience stress or anxiety, their ability to control their eating is likely to be affected, just like stress or anxiety in thin persons will make it more difficult for them to accomplish whatever goals they are pursuing.

When fat people do have emotional problems, they are often related to discrimination, which helps them disparage their bodies and have negative emotional reactions to dieting. Research consistently finds that overweight adolescents and adults have lower self-esteem, lower body-esteem, and see themselves as less attractive than normal weight persons.[32-35] Even those who are not fat but can "pinch more than an inch" consider themselves overweight, diet, feel self-conscious about their bodies, and worry that their social life will be hurt by their excess weight.[36] As society judges overweight women harsher than overweight men, this view is reflected in women's and adolescent girls' self-perception and dissatisfaction with their bodies and a strong desire to lose weight.[8,10] One study in search of disturbance among overweight adolescents failed to find any, except for a greater deal of suppressed anger among the heavier youth compared to normal weight ones.[37] Helpless about society's negative view of them, overweight boys and girls are more likely to have angry feelings that they don't think they should have. After all, it is all their fault . . .

In an effort to gain approval from others, fat persons spend much of their time dieting, which has been found to produce adverse consequences, such as depression, nervousness, weakness, and irritability. Obsession with thinness may also lead to bulimia, particularly in adolescent girls.[10] Once again, these are symptoms that are linked with society's non-acceptance of fatness.

There is nothing intrinsically wrong with the personalities of heavy persons. Being fat, being non-caucasian, being short, or having bad skin all result in some negative outside evaluations. Most of us have some way in which we don't fit societal ideals, and each of us deal with it the best we can. A number of studies looked at people who lost a great deal of weight through gastric stapling. As a result of weight loss patients showed improvement in body image,[38] emotional health,[39] feelings of personal control, and interpersonal functioning.[40] Patients' self-concept improved, they started behaving more assertively and independently, and became more interested in sex with their spouses.[41] On the down side, anxiety and jealousy were prominent among spouses' responses. It is clear that most of their emotional disturbances followed rather than caused their fatness. (Interestingly, being thin brought on its own set of problems, by encouraging anxiety in the formerly fat clients' spouses.)

The stigma leveled against fat people limits their opportunities to develop social skills. They have fewer dates, date fewer persons, and have less sexual involvements than their thinner peers.[34,42] Because they are not as welcomed into social situations, many heavy persons make themselves shy and isolated. Some never develop good social skills, which are normally learned through repeated exposure. Studies of overweight adolescents and adults have found problems in their social interaction.[32] For example, obese young women compared to normal weight women were found to be less able to interpret nonverbal facial cues of males on a videotape.[43] In a study where obese and non-obese women conversed on the telephone with college students who were unaware of the women's weights, judges who were also unaware of the women's weights listened in and rated the women's conversations. Both the judges and the telephone partners rated the obese women as less likable, and as having lesser social skills.[44] This is not surprising in light of the fact that over-weight students spend less time with friends of the other sex than their average weight colleagues.[35]

THE CASE OF MARIA

Maria's history of treatment was one of the most successful and yet disappointing of the many people treated by the authors. She came in to attend a weight loss therapy group and treatment program. She was extremely obese, five feet two inches, 463 pounds and forty-three years old. Despite her size she had a quiet mien of dignity and dressed and presented herself well.

During the first few group sessions Maria spoke very little and even with prompts by the psychologist and the other group members she remained relatively silent. Her weight loss was outstanding, as she lost thirty pounds in the first two weeks. This success had facilitated her willingness to disclose more in the group. The other members were so congratulatory and supportive that she apparently felt she could trust them. Never in her life had she been out with a man, she had never been kissed, nor was ever told anything nice. She lived with her elderly mother who was, except for some superficial acquaintances at work, her only friend. Allowing for her shyness, there was no discernable reason, except her weight, that she would be so alone. Yet, she did not complain or lament. Maria seemed to have accepted her lonely life as the only way it could be for her.

By her sixth visit she had lost sixty-three pounds, and she expressed some excitement at her weighing, because this was the first time in her adult life that she could be under four hundred pounds. Sadly, she gained weight and stayed about the four-hundred-pound barrier. She began to quietly sob and the author was summoned. She was re-weighed, but the scale adamantly stayed on the 404-pound figure. Agony was clearly expressed in her face. The author brought her into a session room. She said she felt doomed. She had nearly starved herself that week and had actually gained weight—it was so unfair. The author explained that body water changes could result in temporary gains, even for people strictly adhering to their dietary regimen. She accepted this explanation but continued on about her suffering as she had not done before. Getting under four hundred pounds was extraordinarily important to her. Three-hundred-pound women were fat but not oddities as she was. She desperately wanted to be normal, she had given up on being attractive or even plain, but she could not bear to be stared at anymore.

Maria explained that years ago she had given up any hope of having a normal life. She had never made love, been kissed by a man, or been on a date. Having ruled out the possibility of such luxuries, she resolved to quietly work, avoid attention and live a simple life. But now for the first time in her adult life she felt some hope. After the impromptu session Maria resolved once again to go back on the dietary program. Over the next eight weeks she did quite well, losing another forty-four pounds, a total of 107 pounds. At this weight, one which most people would consider quite high, Maria began to notice some changes. She had gone from 463 pounds to 356 pounds. She was still fat, but she said that others were treating her better. For the first time in twelve years at her company she was invited to the Christmas party, a positive event that evoked some painful memories. She said that people were now talking to her like a real person, sometimes even giving her compliments.

But to the concern of the therapist and the other members of the group she began to seem increasingly distressed at these exciting changes in her life. She began to complain that these people bothered her and that she didn't know what to say. After some pressure from the group members she went to the company Christmas party. The group members were surprised at her demeanor at the following session. She was sullen and irritable, and more laconic than she had been since she first began. With repeated probing she confessed that she had a terrible time at the party and felt extraordinarily self-conscious. She seemed to think out loud when saying that she wondered if it was worth it. The therapist, with the group's support, chided her on her self-downing, but showed that they accepted *her*, and pushed her to stay with losing some more weight.

She never returned to the group and would not take any calls from the therapist. In further group sessions it became clear from the few discussions that Maria had with other members that she felt awkward, and at a loss with other people. Her isolation had prevented her from mastering the social skills that others take for granted. Her progressive thinness became increasingly frightening, until she decided to give up and stay heavy and isolated.

Self-Control

Perhaps the most frequent accusation that fat people are faced with is that they have "no self-control." But research is clear on the fact that fat persons generally eat no more than thin persons. Thus, lack of self- control is not responsible for their weight. Overeating may be responsible for at most 20–30 pounds of extra body fat, but those who are more overweight than that have a metabolism responsible for their state. Fat persons themselves may testify that they have a hard time controlling themselves around food, but this is because they are constantly dieting, and they are plain hungry. A person of any weight would have a hard time controlling himself around food if he were told to eat dramatically less than what his body naturally craves.

Some overweight persons do indeed have a greater affinity for food, and some may have a hard time controlling their sweet tooth. Certainly, fat persons are not one hundred percent in control of their eating, or of other aspects of their lives. But do thin people have more self-control than fat people? The first problem with this idea is that many thin people have little self-control, which does not show itself in the number of pounds they carry. Weight is not an issue for many, they eat what they want and their body keeps their weight down without any effort. But there are many other ways of being out of control, aside from overeating, that are less obvious to the casual observer. Thin persons may have problems getting to work on time, concentrating on their work, controlling their drinking, smoking, or drugging, controlling their temper, etc. These ways of not being in control are not apparent at first glance, but they can be much more damaging to the individual and those around him or her than overweight is. Fatness on the other hand, is noticed at first glance, and people usually infer that the cause is lack of control around food.

Because social pressure drives almost all of us to desire to be thin, your being fat often shows that you have not as *much* control over your eating as you may want to exert. It does show that you are not one hundred percent in control. But it does not show that you and other fat or chubby people have *less* self-control than do thin people. No one has one hundred percent control, but less than perfect control, and human fallibility, "show" more in fat or chubby people.

For those whose natural setpoint is higher than society's ideal, constant self-denial and strong will-power is necessary to keep the weight under setpoint. A naturally heavy person might decide that keeping her weight down is not worth constant self-denial. This is a perfectly rational option, which does not show weakness, only a decision to enjoy life, as much as her prejudiced society will allow her to enjoy it, without continually depriving herself.

Dieting is not the only way to have willpower and self-control, but it is one way. Socialite Ivana Trump was quoted in 1986 as saying, "It makes me feel powerful to be hungry." Ivana successfully chose to exert control over her hunger. She had will-power in *this* area, though in *other* areas her self-control may have been weaker.

A person who wants to show herself that she has control over her urges, perhaps because of other things in her life, may focus in on her weight and make it a larger issue than just health and good looks—she may make it a moral issue. "If I can control my weight, I am a good, strong person, worthy of love, worthy of a happy future." She may tie up her fatness with her whole life and worth as a human being. Numbers on her scale become a symbolic measure of her "total goodness" or "badness." Now that so much is at stake, she perversely makes her feelings of hunger pleasurable. They are "proof" of moral fiber, proof of her being OK. This is the road to anorexia nervosa (pathological thinness), to never feeling thin enough, to enjoying self-deprivation.

Is absolute control necessary in life? Clearly not, because none of us have it and we are still able to cope. Giving up the demand that you must have total control of your life will free you to accept yourself better, and to use your energies where you can shine, rather than obsessing over whether or not imperfections like "extra" pounds show. Society strongly encourages dieting, but *you* are the only one who can accept its goals and *make yourself* feel worthless. You can watch your weight and still always—yes always—see yourself as a person like everyone else, with skills, talents, and enjoyments.

Notes for Chapter 5.

1. Pollack Seid, 1989.
2. Kleinke & Staneski, 1980.

3. Silverstein, Peterson & Perdue, 1986.
4. Nasser, 1988.
5. Bruch, 1978.
6. Allon, 1973.
7. Harris, 1990.
8. Jasper & Klassen, 1990.
9. Hiller, 1982.
10. Wadden & Stunkard, 1987.
11. Wadden & Stunkard, 1985.
12. Hiller, 1981.
13. Richardson, Goodman, Hastorf & Dornbusch, 1963.
14. Goodman, Donbusch, Richardson & Hastorf, 1963.
15. Maddox, Back & Liederman, 1968.
16. English, 1991.
17. DeJong, 1980.
18. Lerner, 1980.
19. Canning & Mayer, 1966.
20. Pargaman, 1969.
21. Larkin & Pines, 1979.
22. Roe & Eickwort, 1976.
23. Industry Week, 1974.
24. Rothblum, Brand, Miller & Oetjen, 1990.
25. Benson, Severs, Tatgenhorst & Loddengaard, 1980.
26. Jasper & Klassen, 1990.
27. Bellizzi, Klassen & Belonax, 1989.
28. Larkin & Pines, 1979.
29. Crandall & Biernat, 1990.
30. Harris & Smith, 1982.
31. Young & Powell, 1985.
32. Sobal, 1984.
33. Cash & Hicks, 1990.
34. Kallen & Doughty, 1984.
35. Hendry & Gillies, 1978.
36. Tiggemann, 1988.
37. Johnson, 1990.
38. Leon, Eckert, Teed & Buchwald, 1979.
39. Larsen, 1990.
40. Chandarana, Conlon, Holliday & Deslippe, 1990.
41. Marshall & Neill, 1977.
42. Sobal, 1984a.
43. Giannini, DiRusso, Folts & Cerimele, 1990.
44. Miller, Rothblum, Barbour & Brand, 1990.

6

What Weight is Beautiful? (It Depends on Who You Ask.)

"Sick of going from diet to diet, hating myself for not being thin or for yo-yoing from fat to almost-thin-enough, I am surely an inferior creature, an abomination . . . I am not thin, I have fat, I have cellulite. I am disgusting! How could anyone want me? If anyone did want to get near me, I could never let them see me naked. They must not realize how fat and horrible I really am under my clothing. I must hide until (if ever) I get thin . . . "

Does this at all sound like you? Such thoughts are in the minds of many women—obese women, "fat" women, but also women considered "normal weight" by most standards. Many women (and some men) live with a great deal of pain and self-loathing, because they believe that if they do not live up to our beauty standard then by definition they are ugly and unacceptable. Self-condemnation based on the shape of your body is only possible if you fail to see the whole picture—that there is a wide range of human weights and shapes, and you do not have to go by the ideals of one group of people in one era. Even within a society that chooses the "thin, blond" ideal for example, you can make your own choices.

We live in a very visual society, where people spend a great deal of time watching television and movies. One national pastime is watching beauty contests—"Miss America," "Miss U.S.A.," "Mrs. America," "Mr. America," "Miss Universe." Unfortunately, most of the persons on television are above average in attractiveness and style, and viewers forget to remind themselves that most people do not look like the people on TV, in fact even the people themselves do not look that perfect off-screen.

We see women in ads selling toilet-bowl cleaners, caught in the act of cleaning, who look more appealing than most other mere mortals do as they get ready for an evening on the town. Afternoon soap operas purport to present regular people who get caught up in interesting situations, but no one on soap operas looks average.

Television is a powerful image maker. It places a sharp focus on physical beauty as opposed to inner beauty, because that is what it does best—convey images. But is physical beauty as important for having a happy, meaningful life as television might make us believe? Cannot average or even plain looking people excel in many ways, or influence the lives of millions of people?

There is no doubt that presidential candidates have more important attributes than their appearance, but there is also no doubt that voters are greatly influenced by how charming and pleasing to the eye the candidates are. That is why ex-movie stars often have a better chance of becoming elected than persons who have spent their lives in government and who perhaps don't have the same natural good looks.

Appearances are important in day-to-day dealings as well as in presidential elections, because people do make (unfounded) judgments of a person's inner characteristics based on external cues. It is therefore advisable to make the best of your appearance by using good hygiene, wearing fashionable clothes that fit, getting a good hair cut, and otherwise being well groomed. In romantic situations appearance certainly plays a large role. But how perfect must you look? And what is perfect anyway? In this chapter we show you how society changes its definition of beauty and proper weight, and we discuss how important it is for you to fit these changing standards.

A healthy appearance has always been considered beautiful. But, as we've shown in Chapter 1, what a healthy weight is for each individual cannot be easily determined with height-weight charts. While societies have varied from decade to decade on their choices of ideal beauty, because of the uniformity brought on by television, we now are more narrow in our definition of beauty than we were in the 18th century and earlier.

Roberta Pollack Seid reviewed the fashions of the body throughout the ages, finding that, just as fashion in clothing changed, the ideal body changed its size and shape.[1] Thus, the early Greeks believed in balance and moderation and disdained extremes in either direction. One Greek poet wrote about the different kind of wives that a man, if not careful, may be saddled with: "The long haired sow doesn't take baths but sits about in a shift of dirty clothes and gets fatter and fatter." On the other hand, it is also a calamity if she looks like a monkey, "hardly has an ass and her legs are skinny. What a poor wretch is the husband who has to put his arms around such a mess!" Early greek statues depicting Aphrodite show a woman who is not obese, but significantly heavier than our present ideal. The same ideal of plumpness was maintained by the early Roman culture.

The next "beauty trend" was that the body was not fashionable in any form: with the advent of early Christianity, the body was temptation, and was to be concealed with flowing, thick garments. Then during the late Middle Ages and the Renaissance, art resurrected the human body in a variety of shapes. The gothic nude was thin, but different from our ideal: the women were portrayed as short-legged and short-waisted, with protruding stomachs,

sloping shoulders and thin arms. This was a more tradi-
tionally feminine shape, delicate and with emphasis on her
procreative function. Botticelli's Venus during the same
period portrays a more voluptuous shape, though somewhat thinner than the Greek Aphrodite. Other sculptures,
such as the Vanitas, showed even heavier women, "like the
'before' photos in ads for weight loss," as Pollack Seid
notes. She also notes that all these depictions had in
common health and symmetry, in an age where deformities were commonplace. Skin diseases, nutritional deficiencies, fleas and lice, crooked teeth, crippled legs and
arms due to a lack of obstetrical knowledge or accidents
later in life, and little medical knowledge to prevent or
cure all of these defects, made healthy, smooth bodies of
varying weights and shapes beautiful by comparison.

A variety of ideals continued to exist, but the large
female ideal became much larger by the end of the 15th
century as can be seen in the works of Leonardo Da Vinci,
Rubens, and Rembrandt. At the beginning of the 19th
century, Pierre Auguste Renoir was still painting voluptuous nudes. As recently as the turn of the century, one of
the most admired American beauties was the actress Lilian
Russell, weighing two hundred pounds.

Throughout most of human history thinness was considered unattractive, a sign of poverty. Up to the industrial
revolution, food was not easily available and people had to
do hard physical work to obtain it. Fat was admired as a
sign of affluence, showing that a person did not need to
engage in physical labor to earn a living. (Similarly, pale
skin was idealized because only the idle rich could afford to
stay out of the sun.) Anthropologists record that the most
respected tribal chieftains had the fattest pigs and the
fattest wives.[2] For men as well, stoutness was associated
with power, virility, and success.

The preference for plumpness may have developed
partially because it was rare, and therefore valued. Also,
stout women were considered stronger, better able to

carry out chores, and better able to become pregnant and carry a fetus to term. Or perhaps the pretty women in hunting and gathering times became heavier because they were favored by the male hunters and given more to eat.

Statues and paintings throughout the ages clearly show us that heavy women were appreciated through much of history. Fertility goddesses in primitive cultures had large breasts, stomachs, thighs and derrieres. One of the oldest statues, known as Venus of Willendorf, dating back about 20,000 years, has a round figure that would be called morbidly obese today. So were Greek and Roman goddesses depicted. Historians describe Cleopatra, Queen of the Nile, as quite plump.

Overweight is valued today as well, in most parts of the world. In most non-western societies, including but not limited to Third World countries, there is a strong positive relationship between socio-economic status and obesity among men, women, and children. Those who have the good fortune to be able to afford eating a great deal do so, and the weight they gain is admired as a status symbol.[3,4] A recent study surveyed twenty-five contemporary tribal cultures concerning their ideal in female beauty. All but five of the tribes preferred plump to obese women.

Peoples of Third World origins, such as Afro-Americans and Hispanics living in western societies, still look kindly on fatness, and continue to consider slightly overweight (by modern standards) women attractive, even though scarcity of food is no longer a problem. Women have the opportunity to easily become overweight, and they often do so. One study[5] found that among a random sample of adults in the United States almost half of black women were "overweight" by accepted national standards, compared to less than a fifth of white women. Black men were also somewhat heavier than white men. Cultural values accepted these differences in weight. This study also found that most men, black and white, and most black women did not feel that they had a weight problem, whereas among white women all but the ones who were underweight reported that they had a weight problem and wanted to lose weight.[5]

Overweight is not valued in modern western society because it no longer conveys the message that the fat individual is affluent or powerful. Almost anyone can now afford to be fat. In fact, it costs more to be thin. Ten billion dollars are spent yearly on diets, as twenty million Americans are dieting at any moment. Money is spent on diet programs, doctor's bills, lotions to rid the body of cellulite, and potions to decrease appetite. Special diet foods are more expensive—they require more processing. It also costs money to belong to an exercise club or to buy one's own exercise equipment. Time consumption, of course, is expensive.

Research shows that in developed (western) societies, weight decreases with increasing social class, especially for women.[3,4,6,7] For men and children the trend is not quite so strong. There are many reasons why the poor get fatter and the rich get thinner. One reason is that poor persons cannot afford nutritious and less fattening foods and the time for regular exercise. Another reason is natural selection, especially in the case of women. Women who aspire to rise socially try to keep their weight down, and those who succeed in becoming thin have a better chance to improve their station in life. A third reason is that those of lower economic status tend to be minorities, and minorities are more culturally accepting of fatness.

The trimming down of the large voluptuous ideal in western culture culminated, in the '60s, with the "Twiggy era." Seventeen-year-old model Twiggy came to represent the height of fashion in 1967 with a five foot seven and one-half inch frame, weighing a meager ninety-one pounds. In the 1960s thinness took on a meaning in addition to being considered aesthetically pleasing. It meant relinquishing the middle class values of one's middle-aged parents, and becoming perpetually young and free and thin.

We now maintain an appreciation of thinness and the pursuit of youth, though recently there has been a pull away from the "skin and bones" look. A somewhat fuller, somewhat muscular body is now in vogue. One reason is because we are learning about the value of good health apart from size alone. Another reason is that when there is an economic recession there is often a general retreat to "old fashioned" values, which include an appreciation of plumpness as a symbol of prosperity. However, most women are still reluctant to give up the constant vigilance over their food intake to which they've become accustomed. An article in the Living Section of the *New York Times* (January 2, 1991) notes that today "forks are poised somewhere between plate and mouth." Women of fashion are no longer sure whether to "fast or feast," but just to keep on the safe side, they try to maintain their svelte, underweight figures.

Today's models and actresses weigh more than Twiggy, but their weight is still within the thinnest five percent of the population, far below that of the average healthy woman. Ironically, natural selection has chosen us based on how well we can store fat.[8] Because of plagues, wars, unfavorable weather conditions and poor technology, there were periodic food shortages in pre-industrial societies. Those persons who for biological reasons easily stored fat were more likely to survive the food shortages. During the ice age and later in cold climates once again those who had an extra layering of fat were more likely to survive. Society today disdains the very same traits that allowed its ancestors to survive.

If you choose during these times of plenty to go against the grain and attempt to look like our thin ancestors who died out during famines, you choose to fight an uphill battle. The great majority of women must diet and exercise fervently if they aspire to look fashionable. Different people are at their healthiest at different weights, but our media-driven society demands uniformity of appearance. There is a standard of beauty today which is 20–30 pounds thinner than is necessary for good health. Women are being encouraged to reach a weight that is below their natural setpoint. Being underweight is usually not unhealthy, but the constant vigilance required to maintain such a low weight can take its emotional toll.

Choosing to diet and keep below your natural setpoint range may be a good choice, based on what you may have to gain by looking fashionable. But seeing that thinness is only a modern fashion, that thinness was in fact a hazard when food was scarce, it is not rational to put yourself down for being fat or plump. It is not your "fault," it is not even intrinsically bad. It is simply your reality and, in this society and in these times, your appearance is not at the height of fashion. Is that so terrible? Does that make you gross or subhuman? We do not think so.

Fat is the body's way of storing energy and water; it serves as insulation and keeps the body warm. Last but not least, it allows for reproduction to occur. Perhaps having "too much of a good thing" is not to your advantage, but it would serve you well to see fat as a normal, necessary part of your body. It is not disgusting, and you are not disgusting for having it.

Women and Men—The Meaning of Fat, The Importance of Beauty

The changes in standards for thinness and fitness apply to both genders, but there is no question that women are more affected by changes in fashion regarding how their bodies ought to look. In 1826, Brillat-Savarin wrote that for a man it was alright to be lean, but thinness was "a horrible calamity for women: beauty to them is more than life itself, and it consists above all of the round-ness of their forms and the graceful curvings of their outlines".[9] Tastes have changed, and now there is pressure on women to conform to the new thin ideal.

Fat or thin, women have a larger percentage of their body weight in adipose tissue. From birth, girls generally have a higher fat-to-lean ratio than boys and by the pre-pubescent stage they have ten to fifteen percent more fat than boys. This finding applies across geographic and eth-nic boundaries. At puberty, boys' fat to lean ratio decreases to ten to fifteen percent, while girls develop more fat. Approximately twenty-two percent of a girl's body weight must be composed of fat in order for menstruation to occur.

With age, women's bodies continue to naturally store fat. The average woman in her forties or fifties has about thirty-eight percent body fat and has gained about twenty to thirty pounds. Adult women who make themselves excessively lean (ten to fifteen percent less than normal weight), by dieting and/or excessive exercise, are infertile because they stop ovulating. This is an adaptive mecha-nism of the body, because being underweight decreases the chances of a successful pregnancy outcome. Weight gain restores fertility.[10] Too much fat can also inhibit the menstrual cycle and fertility by disturbing the estrogen-progesterone balance. There are individual differences, however, so that a three hundred-pound woman may be fertile. A moderate amount of fat, but not thinness, in-creases fertility.

Fat is at the essence of femininity, it allows human reproduction to occur. Women's greater amount of fat tissue than men's is a natural sex difference, a desirable difference. The extra fat keeps women's skin soft and smooth, unlike men's. Fat is malleable and it allows wom-en's bodies to vary much more than men's. Fat is associ-ated with femininity: warm, soft, comforting, motherly, soft breasts. Hardness is associated with masculinity.

When women gain weight, their femininity is usually ac-centuated: breasts swell and buttocks become enlarged.

We could speculate that the modern taste for thinness may have to do with changes in women's roles within the workforce of our industrialized society. A total rejection of fat in women is equivalent to a rejection of womanhood. With the industrial revolution and with the women's movement, women have found that being seen as very feminine, and very different from men, can be costly in a society where men are held as the standard in the work arena. When women become thinner they become more angular, more like men, giving the illusion that they can do the job, *because* they appear similar to males. However, by making oneself thinner and more masculine, women in the long run adopt a self- defeating strategy, bound to keep them in an inferior position. "Masculinized" women may be accepted in the workforce more readily, but they will never be equals if they are to be judged solely on their ability to be "like men." Women, on the average, will always be less masculine than men. If they reject their femininity, they are ultimately accepting an inferior status. They are in effect saying "I know I was born with this handicap of being female, but I will overcome it!"

Our present concern with physical good looks is actu-ally the result of a prosperous lifestyle. We can now (in some classes in some parts of the world) afford the luxury of not only surviving, but seeking more aesthetically pleasing surroundings, including attractive friends and lovers. Up to the 18th century, arranged marriages were the norm, and the primary considerations were economic and social standing of the two mates. Estates, fortunes, and noble pedigrees were passed on to new families in this manner. In the lower social classes as well, marriages were arranged according to what each partner could bring into the part-nership. Especially for girls, the size of their dowry largely determined their chances for a good husband. Physical appearance was not important for marriage, though it played a role in men's choice of mistresses and, to a smaller extent, in married women's choice of lovers. Beauty was always appreciated, but it only played a small role in determining one's social standing.

In the 18th century, romantic love came to be in vogue; defying one's parents' wishes, eloping with an "inappropriate" but enticing love choice. Young girls now had to attract their mates with their beauty and charm. Men became more able to gain resources without resorting to unwanted marriages. They could now afford to "purchase" beauty as well as material possessions. This trend strengthened with the advent of capitalism, in which old titles and old money are no longer essential for social standing or for acquiring wealth. However, because women as a group are less financially well off than men (partially because of fewer opportunities and lower pay and partially because they spend a significant proportion of their time and energy on child rearing), they still look for economic security in a spouse more than men do.

Up to very recently, men have seldom tried to lose weight solely to improve their appearance. When they have dieted, they did so primarily for health reasons. Their appearance has not been as much equated with their overall worth as women's. In patriarchal societies, where men owned property and controlled finances, women gained economic security by trading in their physical appeal for financial support. They most likely preferred good-looking men, but could not afford to be very choosy, as their first priority was financial security.

Today this picture has changed somewhat, as most women work and can support themselves. They now have more "bargaining chips"—their own incomes and positions as well as their appearance. Perhaps in direct response to this shift, men have become more looks- and weight-conscious themselves. Men no longer had better disregard their appearance!

But women still make significantly fewer dollars per

hour than men, and the task of raising children is a difficult one for a woman alone. Men are still needed to help out financially. Further, that there are still more adult women than men. Their scarcity makes men more desirable, so once again they have more "bargaining chips," and less incentive to worry about perfecting themselves in order to please women.

> "To men, a man is but a mind. Who cares what face it carries? Or what form he wears? But a woman's body *is* the woman."
>
> —Ambrose Bierce[11]

To most men, a woman's appearance is of utmost importance in determining romantic interest. Research and just casual observation of male habits (reading "girlie" magazines, frequenting bars with go-go dancers, watching pornography films) shows that men get sexually excited from visual stimuli more than do women. Further, being seen with a beautiful woman and driving an expensive car are perhaps the two greatest symbols of being a successful male in this society. Consequently, women's appearance determines to a large extent their success with men. Among 514 personal ads, 56.9 percent of males specified that they desired a physically attractive female, while only 26.4 percent of the woman ad writers specified physical attractiveness as a prerequisite.[12]

One-third of the males in this study also stated a weight preference (e.g. slim, thin, or petite woman wanted), while hardly any (only two percent) of the women stated a weight preference. Women do have preferences, e.g. for the tall thin ascetic type, the "teddy bear" type, the Apollo type, but they are less concerned with physical shape.

Weight (i.e., thinness) has been found to influence the number of responses women receive to personal ads they place[13] and the number of weekly dates that women, but not men, report.[14] There is some question, however, about how thin is "in." Research shows that men want their women to be heavier than women like themselves to be, while women like men to be thinner than men like themselves to be.[15]

Overall, women have bought the thin ideal more than men. In fact, it is fair to say that a large proportion of contemporary women are obsessed with thinness. This irrational demand for slenderness at all costs has many roots, societal, and perhaps biological as well. Women are indeed given the message that they *are* their bodies. Women define their self-worth in terms of winning approval and having a pleasing appearance, while men largely judge themselves by their accomplishments. Whether or not you choose to accept society's values, your disturbance stems from your absolutistic demands. As a woman, you foolishly convince yourself that you *must* be gorgeous and thin even if you have to starve yourself and spend all your money on plastic surgery. You wrongly think that you *must* get approval, love, and admiration from all those who matter, or else you are worthless, unfeminine, and hardly human. If you are a man, you take society's goal that you'd *better* succeed and change it to "I *must* succeed in business or my profession, even at the cost of high blood pressure and heart attacks."

The *preference* to be beautiful, thin, popular or successful is quite rational—we all want the good things in life. But it is also rational to realize that we cannot have all the good things we prefer. Fully realizing this is liberating, because it will give us permission to be imperfect, to have frustrations in life. We don't really *need* to be outstanding at everything we do, and we don't *need* everyone's approval. If, for example, a moderately overweight woman has a husband who finds her attractive and has a job that she likes, she can choose to upset herself and put herself down over her weight, or she can choose to accept her weight and her metabolism, and enjoy what in fact is a good life.

For us to have a *preference* as opposed to a *demand* usually means assessing the pros and cons of a situation and trying to reach a preferred state, instead of tying in our self-worth with something that is often not under our control. Later in this book we talk about self-acceptance and acceptance of disadvantageous situations, which frees you to determinedly and steadily work at making the best of a situation, and frees your mind from obsessing about what could have been, what "should" have been.

Women's irrational demands may be even more pernicious than men's, because the things they demand are less under their control. Men may irrationally demand that they "must" be successful at all costs, but this is a state they can often achieve with hard work, and can objectively measure by their title, salary and other rewards. Women's "success," on the other hand, is at the mercy of others. "Others" must find them attractive and nice. Beauty is in the eye of the beholder, and the beholder holds the key to many women's sense of self-worth. When is a woman attractive *enough*? Physical flaws accumulate with age, with bearing children. When is a woman nice *enough*? Can she ever please everyone? If she cannot, is she obviously a *bad person*?

Driven by the irrational *need* to please and to be loved, many women become obsessed with thinness and carry their slenderness to extremes that most men would not even find appealing.[14-16] Perhaps because weight is easier to adjust than one's features, the scale becomes the symbolic battleground—the way to liking oneself and hopefully being liked by all.

Weight is easier to change than your height, but it is not infinitely malleable, as you may hope. The way fat distributes itself on your body is genetically determined. Just try to change it!

Women are frequently unhappy about their particular shape—about their breasts, waistline, or thighs somehow deviating from their ideal. One common complaint was labeled the "violin deformity" by a Toronto newspaper.[17] This "deformity" consists of the midhip being narrower than the "love handles" above it, and the "thunder thighs" below it, rather than having one smooth curve from waist to knee. About seventy-five percent of all women have some approximation of this "deformed" shape. How can the most common body type be considered a deformity? Only by using extremist "black and white" thinking, by demanding perfection, and by overlooking the reality staring us in the face. If three quarters of the female population has a certain shape, it is by definition a normal shape, not a deformity. Perhaps it is not the most beautiful shape we could conceive of, but its prevalence makes it normal by any reasonable judgment. It is cruel and unusual punishment for women to be held to such a high standard of appearance that most of them will feel deformed and many will hate themselves for being "deformed."

The article about the "violin deformity" was, not surprisingly, written by a woman. It is mainly women who hold themselves to such high standards of thinness. Men's tastes in women are somewhat different, and can be discerned from the magazines they peruse. In X-rated magazines used by men solely for masturbation, the women portrayed are more voluptuous and curvaceous than the thin ideal. While many men say that they don't like fat women, thinness is not what they particularly find attractive. Most men are attracted to feminine attributes that they themselves don't have: to breasts and to buttocks that expand from the waist. If women would only note and accept this reality, they would be more accepting of themselves and their bodies.

Individual preferences vary a great deal, often clashing with that which is considered societally acceptable. Many men are sexually attracted to very overweight women.

THE CASE OF BONNIE

Bonnie had just turned thirty-two when she saw one of the authors for help with her weight problem. Her obesity was such that it was her most defining feature. At five foot seven inches and 332 pounds, Bonnie appeared quite large. Exacerbating her excessive weight was her dress and demeanor. She wore a loose fitting and unflattering tunic-like dress, used little or no makeup and had close cropped hair, which gave her the appearance of a chubby adolescent boy. Her demeanor was as uncomplimentary as her apparel and grooming. She sat facing the author hunched forward with her arms around her abdomen. She was clearly anxious and very self-conscious. Bonnie seemed desperate and scared as she told her story.

She had been fat as far back as she could remember, and all her memories centered around the abuse she received as a result of it. Starting as a young girl, and from then on, she was told she was wasting her attractive face by being so fat. She was asked by family, teachers and her few friends why she stayed that fat. Of course, she had no idea *why* she was fat, but she became increasingly certain everyone disliked her. Her rage was plain when she told of her third grade physical education teacher telling her she was too fat to play punch ball with the other girls. Even the school nurse told her to lose weight as though she was being told to change clothes. Bonnie had no concept of how to lose weight, although she did know that eating made her feel good.

Her parents brought her to her family physician who put her on an exchange diet. This served only as another source of pain as her slender younger sister would have another reason to mock her as both fat *and* weak. Her physician then gave her diet pills. She became agitated and distressed while taking the pills but, as with previous diets, she lost very little weight.

The diet attempts continued, but so too did the suggestions from all the significant people in her life for new ways to lose. It seemed to Bonnie that no one could talk to her without attacking her about her weight. Everyone was thinking about her being fat and was out to hurt her. Her solution was to withdraw from people. She became increasingly hostile.

This style had become an essential part of Bonnie's personality by the time she came in for treatment. Psychological testing evidenced that she suffered from anti-social, paranoid, and passive-aggressive personality disorders. Many sessions would begin with Bonnie, wearing a Cheshire cat grin, saying with mock concern, "I'm really in trouble." She would follow with tales of shop-lifting, vandalism, or acts of pure cruelty.

As a result, she was placed in both group and individual therapy and put on a very restrictive diet. She seemed to come alive in the group, as though she had found her place in the world. Always smiling broadly she would gleefully report her rapid and consistent losses to the group. Her individual sessions were not quite as straightforward. She struggled against her paranoid style and her continual anger. She stubbornly held the belief that most people hated her because she was fat and that she had to have their approval or they would hate her more. So she smiled and made small talk with everyone she would meet in the office, while carefully registering every nuance of their speech and behavior as potential slights and insults directed at her.

At the eighteenth week of treatment Bonnie had dropped to 228 pounds. She had lost more than five pounds per week, and had never lost less than three pounds in any week on the diet. Weight loss this rapid and consistent had only been observed in clients who demonstrated signs of compulsive eating or

bingeing behaviors. That is, those people who became obese solely from excessive eating always
seemed to lose the fastest. Although she was still
more than seventy pounds away from her goal, Bonnie looked strikingly improved. She began wearing
make-up, bought several fashionable dresses, and appeared significantly more confident.

At her private session Bonnie announced she had
been introduced to a man by another member of the
weight group and had dated him twice. She was
almost euphoric, but at the same time she was concerned that he might not be good enough. Bonnie's
self-downing led to the logic "any man who would
want me must have something wrong with him." For
the next few weeks they began seeing each other
regularly. At thirty-three years of age, this was the
first relationship she had ever had with a man; and, as
it turned out, her first sexual experience. The relationship continued for several weeks and Bonnie began attending the group sessions less and less frequently. She began to complain during her individual
sessions that she felt overly deprived on the diet and
needed more food. She expanded her diet, refocused
on her new relationship, and gradually began to gain
weight back.

Her first love affair ended within three months,
but he was replaced with a man from the weight
therapy group. Her attendance was regular, but she
proceeded to progressively gain. This relationship
lasted a bit longer than the first, but ended with
Bonnie just a bit under three hundred pounds. She
stated that she felt out of control and seemed to look
for someone to blame for her relapse. She blamed her
therapist for not letting her eat solid food sooner (she
was on a liquid nutritional supplement diet), and for
not being supportive enough. She blamed her lovers
for upsetting her. She failed to develop the resolve to

get back to her goal of losing the weight. Instead, she dropped out of the therapy group and expanded her social life. Bars and social clubs became a nightly affair. Although professing a desire to be thinner, she seemed to be satisfied with her new sociable lifestyle. Sadly, her weight continued upward. After six months, she had gained all but ten pounds of her original weight back.

Surprisingly, even though she was, once again, more than double her goal weight, she now had no difficulty in finding male companionship. Session after session she would describe men who importuned her company. And more often than not she took up their offers. In individual sessions she would sometimes express concern at her active sexual lifestyle, but the concern was not deep or painful. She thrived on the attention. Her lovers usually were men from less developed countries, which had not labeled obesity as loathsome. Some of the men who sought her attentions actually were married or involved with women who were slender, but found her large size compelling. Bonnie, no doubt, had a talent for communicating her availability, but this did not explain her success. It revealed that there were many men who found her sexually attractive.

Her desirability to these men overcame society's fiat against men being seen with an obese woman. She had sexual relationships with eight men over the next year. Most of these were limited to sexual contacts. One actually involved a taxi driver who would pick her up in his cab to have a brief sexual liaison. He never took her out or acknowledged having a relationship with her. She said she didn't mind this because he was very attractive, and she liked her ability to sexually excite him. According to Bonnie he had a slim, attractive girlfriend with whom he lived. This seemed to make things even more exciting for her.

After all, he had his girlfriend and was still attracted to her! After many sessions that focused on the beliefs that provoked Bonnie's anger, she began to focus on her flawed philosophy of life that made consistent behavior in any area of life difficult. She began to understand that she viewed the world as very hostile. From this global view came her irrational Beliefs such as: "I must keep on my guard all the time," "If someone wrongs me (or appears to have wronged me) I absolutely must get back at them," "If anyone finds out about me I will be destroyed because my secrets are so shameful," and "I must get the goods on others, before they get them on me."

Although the understanding of her irrationality did not produce any sudden or magical changes in Bonnie's deeply deviant personality, it helped her begin a process that continued until this writing. She obtained a job working with people and was able to maintain it for an extended period of time. She also expanded her social life and reduced the amount of her interpersonal hostility.

Society's standards, however, do affect those men who admire very large women. They are often ridiculed, seen as perverse, suffering from neurotic fetishes, or having low self-esteem. Men who are erotically and romantically attracted to fat women sometimes stay "in the closet" about their preference. Society's stigma against men's having sexual alliances with fat women often lead them to disregard their preference, and to marry a thin and fashionable woman, in order to gain social status and peer approval. Consequently, Bonnie will not only have to continue working on her own emotional and interpersonal blocks. She will also have to face rejection even from men who find her sexually appealing. Being very heavy is clearly not preferable for a woman (or a man) in this society.

There is truth to the old saying "You can never be too

rich or too thin." The thinner a woman is, the more likely she is to move into a higher social class, by marriage or otherwise.[18,19] Obese women are more likely to move to a lower socio-economic class than to a higher one.[19]

Notes to Chapter 6.

1. Pollack Seid, 1989.
2. Chase, 1981.
3. Sobal & Stunkard, 1989.
4. Ross & Mirowsky, 1983.
5. Rand & Kuldau, 1990.
6. Whitelaw, 1971.
7. Hendry & Gillies, 1978.
8. Brown & Konner, 1987.
9. Brillat-Savarin, 1926.
10. Frisch, 1988.
11. Bierce, 1983.
12. Smith, Waldor & Trembath, 1990.
13. Lynn & Shurgot, 1984.
14. Stake & Lauer, 1987.
15. Rozin & Fallon, 1988.
16. Zellner, Harner & Adler, 1989.
17. Holub, 1987.
18. Elder, 1969.
19. Goldblatt, Moore & Stunkard, 1992.

7

Origins of Appetite: Physiological, Cultural and Cognitive

As psychologists, we not only seek to treat emotional and life problems but to understand why and how people (and other living things) do the things they do. In the case of eating this is not very difficult. Throughout time the prime goal of humans has been the procurement, preparation and consumption of food. The literature of every human civilization devotes a great deal of space to edibles. We have sacrificed food to the gods, or we drink wine on the holy days, eat of the host, and define certain foods as sacred or reserved for the religious feasts.

If cultures and religions are not focusing on what and how to eat, they are fasting to demonstrate moral or spiritual superiority. The feasts and fasts of Ramadan, the fasting of Yom Kippur, the Friday fast, the privations of Buddha, those who starve themselves to make a political declaration, are prominent examples. It is the unusual social event that does not involve food as a feature. Attendance at a sporting event seems incomplete if one does not eat. Popcorn at movies, hors d'oeuvres at parties, buffets at professional meetings, feasts on saint's days, and peanuts at bars are just a few examples of the intimate connection between specific food and social events. All elucidate the vital role of food as a central focus of human existence.

The complex social role food plays makes it difficult to distinguish its biological importance. Clearly, people eating at social events are not all eating because of a biological drive. Despite the association between obesity and gluttony, you only need to watch people at some of the functions mentioned above to see that virtually all of them will eat with or without an actual physical hunger. But what is hunger? How do we know when the craving for food is based on an actual shortage of a nutrient, or a result of being in a situation that is intimately associated with eating? The answer is that it is indeed very hard to know. In order to understand why and how much we eat, let us examine the biological and psychological aspects of hunger.

Hunger and Appetite

We never question the fact that our bodies are quite capable of regulating our temperatures, our breathing rate, and our fluid balance. We do not assume, for example, that if someone keeps drinking water they are doing so because they have an emotional conflict and they are using the water to drown their troubles. The most common interpretation would be that a drinker has become dehydrated, through exercise or illness, and has developed a physiological craving for fluids. Similarly, if someone is breathing rapidly and short of breath, our first reaction would not be to conclude that they are anal retentive and are compulsively acquiring air. Even a medically naive person who observes someone in this condition would wonder about her having a cardio-pulmonary disorder. Yet when it comes to food consumption we assume that our drive to eat is largely voluntary and psychologically based. However, just as in other appetitive behaviors, such as cravings for air, water, and sex, are partly based on complex biological feed-back mechanisms, the same is true for hunger pangs.

Perhaps we view hunger differently because of the

vast differences we observe in the quantities of food people eat and their body weights. We see such huge differences in both these areas that we tend to conclude that hunger can't possibly be biologically regulated. After all, the brain regulates body temperature and we all center around 98.6 degrees. Why then, if our brains automatically regulate our eating and weight, are there so many individual differences? The answer is that one temperature works best for everybody, but one weight does not fit all. Nevertheless, our body weight is largely a function of our biology, and so is our hunger, our drive to eat.

The experience of hunger is as much a personal phenomenon as the experience of the color red. We really do not know what hunger feels like for another person. For this reason it seems unproductive to try to distinguish hunger types. The simplest defintion is: it is the desire to eat. For most of human history it was assumed that hunger originated in the stomach, when it was empty it conveyed a sense of urgency for food, and when it was full it signaled us to stop eating. This model was simple and fit the personal perception of most people. After all, everyone has heard their stomach growl when empty, and most have felt the distress when it is filled to capacity.

History of Hunger

Walter B. Cannon[1] tested this hypothesis by having a subject swallow a ballon and then monitoring his perception of hunger and his actual stomach contractions. The initial results of these experiments revealed that there was a strong association between the contractions and pressure on the stomach walls. But since Cannon's time hunger has been revealed to be far more complex than pressures on the stomach. Expansion and contraction of the stomach does play a role in feelings of hunger but people without stomachs still get hungry.[1] More recently, placing a ballon in the stomach was touted as a technique of weight reduction, but only produced temporary blocking of hunger.[2,3] Apparently people with a ballon inserted in their stomachs feel less hungry for about two months, and they eat less and lose some weight. After this, however, their hunger mechanisms seem to figure out that their satiety is illusory, the ballon stops working, and their usual hunger returns.

The human body has many redundant systems within it. We have two kidneys, eyes, lungs and so on. In general if some behavior or physical function is critical for survival we generally have back-ups. Hunger is essential. Without motivating forces driving us to eat we humans would have died out eons ago. Early humans typically had to confront grave perils to obtain food, and so their motivating force had to be robust and intense. Given its primary importance, it is not surprising that hunger is at least as multifaceted as other body functions. That is, there had to be more to hunger than the stomach.

The idea that the body has a lipostat, a system that strives to maintain a specific fat proportion, was proposed by G.W. Kennedy. According to this model, hunger will occur when fat levels begin to decline. That is, losing weight will tend to make you feel hungry! This notion has been corroborated in recent studies which demonstrated that fat cells actively seek to keep from being depleted.[4] One study showed that during weight loss, when fat cells begin to empty, they release an enzyme called lipoprotein lipase that both facilitates new fat production, and also increases craving for fatty foods.[5] Just as changes in your weight can result in fat cravings, your genes can also be, at least partially, responsible for your cravings for sweets. Like humans, rats have a marked preference for sweet foods. This predilection for sweets can be increased or diminished by selective breeding. That is, if you take a male rat with a sweet tooth and breed it with a female with a similar preference you are likely to obtain offspring with an even greater desire for sweets.[6] This does not quite prove that we humans inherit our eating propensities from our parents, but it does provide evidence in that direction.

Current Views

Research has demonstrated that the experience of hunger originates from many sources. The human body monitors its levels of several nutrients, and changes in almost any one of them can make us feel hungry. One particularly important food is sugar. Physiologist Jean Mayer first developed the blood sugar theory of hunger.[7] He proposed that variations in blood sugar, in the form of glucose, are responsible for hunger sensations. When blood glucose is high, typically after a meal, we will feel a sense of satiety. After a period of abstinence when our glucose levels have declined we tend to feel increasingly hungry. This theory has been supported by the research which shows that cells in the hypothalamus are sensitive to glucose as well as insulin. This explains why untreated diabetics are frequently hungry despite high blood sugar levels. Insulin facilitates the passage of the blood glucose into the cells. Without it the blood can be full of glucose, but the individual cells can go hungry. When the hypothalamus cells of the diabetic have used all of their available glucose, he or she will experience a desire to eat, despite his high blood sugar levels. Because research has demonstrated that insulin does indeed pass into the brain through capillaries[8] we can conclude that it has the capacity to act directly in the brain. Insulin is not the only hormone that has a direct effect on hunger and appetite. Sex steroids, glucagon, and human growth hormone have been proven to have an effect on increasing appetite.[9,10]

The amount of body fat itself evidently plays a role in hunger. Specifically, the more body fat one has the hungrier one becomes. Animal studies[11-14] have shown that animals who were made fatter on very high-fat diets for prolonged periods of time tended to stay fatter and to eat more than animals who were not fattened in this way. The high-fat diets served not only to increase the *number* of the fat cells (hyperplastic), but the size too (hypertrophic). Perhaps as significant is the fact that animals who had large amounts of fat surgically removed typically began to eat considerably less. This creates the basis of a potential vicious circle, where fat begets more fat.

The liver plays a key role in the processing of fats and it is not surprising that liver function and liver enzymes play a role in hunger.[15] So do the intestines. The gut-peptide cholescystekinin (CCK), which is released during digestion[16,17] plays a role in suppressing hunger. Other peptides found in the body[18,19] can be manipulated to significantly alter hunger. For example, researchers who injected neuropeptide Y into the brains of rats discovered that they doubled their eating, tripled the body fat levels and increased six-fold the rate of weight gain.[20]

Pharmacology and Hunger

For at least a century people have used a broad array of substances to help control their eating. It is not surprising that so many substances have an effect on appetite. With all the endogenous substances—hormones, neurotransmitters, neuromodulators, peptides, etc.—that are involved in the regulation of eating, it is logical that many substances can also interfere with it. Unfortunately, very few of these substances have had a significant long-term effect on body weight. The control of hunger includes a complex number of redundancies. If one systems fails to signal hunger, another will start to do so. You will find it hard to fool your body for any length of time. For shorter periods there are some substances that do seem to help.

The class of drugs that have the most consistent influence on appetite are those that operate on the brain's serotonergic system. Serotonin, or 5-HT, is a neurotransmitter largely associated with brain centers controlling emotions and sleep. The amino acid tryptophan is the primary precursor for the brain's synthesis of serotonin. If the amount of tryptophan that passes into the brain increases, so too will brain levels of serotonin. Consuming carbohydrates[21] encourages the passage of tryptophan into the brain, thereby increasing serotonin production. Serotonin is active in the appetite control centers of the hypothalamus[22-24] which explains part of its role in the control of eating.

In addition to serotonin's role in other brain functions, an increased level is linked to appetite suppression. Tryptophan will pass readily into the brain when carbohydrates are consumed. Because it is a constituent of many proteins, a meal of starch with a minimum of protein will tend to elevate brain serotonin. The brain then uses this neurotransmitter as an appetite regulator. When brain serotonin increases, the appetite centers "conclude" that carbohydrates were consumed.[25,26] So if you were to eat a large meal of pasta, the tryptophan in your blood stream would pass more efficiently into your brain. Your brain would then produce more serotonin, and your craving for carbohydrates would be diminished.

Drugs which elevate brain levels of serotonin have been proven to be quite effective in suppressing eating. One such drug is fluoxetine (Prozac). This drug was developed as an anti-depressant and was subsequently found to have appetite suppressant effects, most notably for carbohydrates.[27-29] Unlike many other anti-depressants which are associated with increased eating, fluoxetine appears to selectively inhibit intake of carbohydrates. It works by selectively blocking the re-uptake of serotonin. Popular wisdom holds that many people self-medicate against depression with chocolates or other candies. This might be an accurate observation based the results of research with fluoxetine.

Dexfenfluramine is another drug that increases brain levels of serotonin. It also is a potent suppressor of eating, most notably carbohydrates. One study found it reduced carbohydrate intake by forty percent. Its close relative, fenfluramine,[30] which has long been used as a diet medication is less selective on which appetites it suppresses. Like amphetamine diet pills, fenfluramine produces more of a central stimulation, and it produces more of a generalized anorexia. Interestingly, dexfenfluramine has been demonstrated[31] to actually decrease the perceived pleasantness of sweets in both obese and non-obese experimental subjects. This tends to corroborate the idea that even food preferences—such as the proverbial "sweet-tooth"—are a function of innate processes.

Naloxone and naltrexone are medications that are used as antidotes for overdoses of opiate drugs, like heroin and morphine. Opiates and narcotics act by binding themselves to positions on the ends of nerve cells that are uniquely suited to receive them. The reason why many of our nerve cells have specific sites on their surfaces that bind with narcotics is because narcotics are molecularly similar to drugs that are naturally found in the brain. These are called endorphins or endogenous morphines.

Endorphins, like the opiate drugs that mimic them, tend to increase eating. This phenomenon can be observed in narcotic addicts who tend to lose their desire to eat when not intoxicated. The addiction seems to disrupt parts of the hunger regulatory system. There is some research to suggest that obese[32-34] people generate greater quantities of endorphins while, and after, eating. The higher level of the brain's own narcotics in obese people seems unrelated to emotional state,[35] or depression; instead it seems to be a basic trait of these individuals. People who report bouts of intense, uncontrollable hunger appear to have especially strong connections between their brain's endorphins and their appetite.[36] When they are given naltrexone they both lose weight and gain greater control of their eating. In fact, a single morning injection of naloxone[37] not only was found to reduce eating, but it also diminished people's thinking about food and their feelings of hunger. The appetite suppression effect of naloxone worked for all food types: proteins, starches and fats.[38]

The tendency of obese people to generate greater

quantities of endorphins may serve to increase weight in two ways. First, it may make ingestion more positively reinforcing, because obese people in effect may get an eater's "high." Second, it may result in a longer period of eating because the euphoria of eating would block or slow the feedback mechanisms that signal people to stop eating. The research indicates that the difference in endorphin functioning is a cause instead of a result of obesity. Obese people who have lost weight continue to show differences in their endorphin functioning.[33]

Substances that show promise in the treatment of obesity and eating control disorders include those substances that the body produces to regulate appetite. Among these are several neuropeptides involved in appetite inhibition, but histidylprolinediketopiperazine also known as cyclo(HisPro) is one of the most potent.[39] It reduces appetite for twelve hours in rodents, inhibits weight gain for up to two weeks, and has potential use in the control of obesity.

The preceding overview further demonstrates the complexity of the physiological mechanisms that regulate body weight and appetite. The fact that many disparate chemicals have major effects on our food behavior indicates that there are many brain and body systems involved in our feeding behavior. It also implies that it is very unlikely that any one drug or medicine will solve the difficulties that dieters face when trying to reduce their weight.

Cognitive Aspects of Hunger

Think back to a time in which you cut your finger or your hand. You probably felt a sharp pain. You looked at it and, to your marked displeasure, noted a nasty gash. You then had thoughts such as, "I cut my finger, I'm bleeding, this is terrible." "What if I can't stop bleeding or need stitches? . . ." Suddenly your finger began to hurt a lot

more intensely, your anxiety further increased, and the
pain became overwhelming.

What happened in a case like this is that your cognitive appraisal of the cut accentuated the intensity of your
pain. If you had been in a life-threatening situation, you
might very well not have noticed the cut at all. In the latter
case, your cognitions would have exclusively focused on
the threat to your life and the pain would have not been
sufficient to produce any significant distress.

Thus, your total experience of pain includes the sensation of the cut, your visual image, your emotion (anxiety,
anger, and rage), your cognitions, and your evaluations.
Consequently, a practical approach is for you to view
hunger as mild pain when you diet. When this pain inten-
sifies, your emotional response may be anxiety, stemming
from your irrational cognitive response, "It will never end,
and I will not be able to stand it!" Research has demonstrated that the anxiety that ensues from your expectation
that the pain of hunger will only get worse leads to dietary
slips. One common result of eating less than you want is
that it hurts. Hunger is painful.

If you are hungry you are in a state of distress. Success
in eating less means that you will have to overcome a
period of personal suffering. A great danger during this
period is your overwhelming belief that, during this difficult time, your distress will never end. If you believe that a
period of suffering is not going to end, you will tend to give
up. On the other hand, you can overcome almost any
suffering if you are able to contemplate it ending. It is your
failure to recognize that the worst hunger pains are temporary that commonly leads you to stop dieting. You can
forget about sincere help from most of your friends and
family because they have never been through this ordeal.
Nearly all people who are not fat believe that if they can be
slender without pain, then fat people should find it equally
easy to become thin. So you suffer alone, without appreciation, consolation, or solace. What you can do, is to help

yourself by challenging your self-defeating thoughts, supplanting them with rational ones, such as these:

"If I don't eat right now, I will continue to lose."

"This one extra food will not really make me feel any better, but it will directly delay my goal."

"The hunger I am feeling is a type of pain. It will fade if I can just wait a half hour. I'll be able to make it."

"The grumbling in my stomach, the empty feelings and the cravings for food *mean I am losing weight*."

"This feeling is temporary, and if I can hold out just an hour or so it will be a major accomplishment!"

"This is the most difficult effort I will ever have to make, and it's worth doing!"

"What will it really do for me if I eat now? I will still want food but will have to work even harder to lose weight."

"How will I feel if I give in to the pain? (Think back to the previous times when you have given in, during other weight-loss attempts)."

"Will my peers, friends and loved ones respect me if I give in to their sabotage or discouragement?"

"How will I feel if I hold out a bit longer?"

"If I've done it for a few days why can't I do it for as long as it takes; how is now different?"

Rational self-statements and questions like these will remind you that most painful feelings are temporary. When you forget that they are temporary, you almost always give in and give up dieting. If you can get yourself to hold off from self-defeating behaviors, even for a short time, your probability of long-term success has increased.

This is an important, yet subtle point. Always remember that even if you fail in any one situation, if you make the extra and ongoing effort you will succeed in the long term. That is, you can *always* try. It is this continued effort that will pay off.

If you recall that most pain, even severe pain, tends to diminish with time, disputing your irrational beliefs will get you through. Your coping statement, "This discomfort is only temporary and I *can* stand it!" will frequently offset your irrational belief that the discomfort of dieting will never end.

Losing Weight: What to Expect

You can alter your weight by consuming fewer or more calories, but there is not a simple relationship between these two plans. Your body is unique in the way it metabolizes food. According to the setpoint theory, borne out by numerous animal and human studies, there is a range within which your body feels comfortable: you don't have to force yourself to eat to reach that range, and you don't have to starve yourself either. Your setpoint ranges within ten percent to fifteen percent of your weight. The high end of your setpoint is likely to be the highest weight you've ever reached. When you reach that high end, you can comfortably eat as much as you want and not gain weight. Even if you forced yourself to overeat, you would only gain a little weight, and it would easily come off as soon as you stopped over-feeding yourself.

Some people's setpoints are above average, others' below. We have seen poignant examples of the rigidity with which setpoints can keep people within certain boundaries in some of our clients who were very thin and were trying to gain weight. Their efforts made them less successful than most of our weight loss clients.

Setpoints themselves can and do change, but unfortunately they usually change in an undesired direction—

they become higher. Eating a constant number of calories, adult women on the average can expect to gain one pound a year. Keeping the weight down becomes more difficult with age. Some women find it hard to lose weight after giving birth, because their bodies have settled into a higher weight.

The good news is that if you eat *everything you want*, you will not keep on gaining weight, but will stabilize at a certain point. Most dieters would be afraid to try this as an experiment, but we do know it to be a fact from research findings. It would seem like an ideal situation, eating as much as you want and not gaining weight, except for the facts that the high end of most people's setpoint is higher than what is considered ideal in this society. Also, health issues are a concern in some cases. Especially for men whose increased pounds mainly settle on the stomach, which is associated with heart disease.

To determine the range of your setpoint, subtract ten to fifteen percent of your present weight. If you are now 200 pounds, the lower end of your setpoint is between 170 and 180 pounds. So if you are now at your highest weight of two hundred pounds and would like to lose twenty or thirty, research shows that you can do that without extremely depriving yourself. In the following chapters we help you gain control over your eating by becoming aware of your eating patterns and your motivations behind them, and by finding more rational ways of thinking about and dealing with food.

If you prefer, however, to be 150 pounds, be prepared for your body to put up much more of a fight against your achieving this. If you would look most appealing to most people at 150 pounds and you are now two hundred, you have been unlucky in your genetic inheritance. You and your genes may help humanity survive in times of famine, but here in the 20th century in Western society, most people will not appreciate your chubby genes, and the only way you can gain their approval is by vigilantly and continuously depriving yourself of the nourishment your body will keep demanding. Yes, deprive yourself to take off weight, and continue depriving yourself to keep it off.

Diet books mention "plateaus" in dieting, where, after having lost some of the weight and still sticking to the same regimen, you are no longer losing. This happens for two reasons. The first reason is most commonly given, but it does not present the full story: at a lower weight you need fewer calories to maintain that weight, and even fewer calories to reduce, so that the number of calories you started to diet with may be too high. However, most diet regimens are around one thousand calories or less per day, an amount at which you should be able to lose weight even if, for example, you went from two hundred pounds to 170.

The second reason for plateaus in weight reduction, which is more supported by research, is that your body is fighting back. You have reached or are about the reach the lower end of your setpoint, and your body is quickly learning to metabolize every bit of food you take in more efficiently, so that it can maintain a weight at which it is comfortable. (Visualize thousands of shrunken, deprived fat cells, screaming for replenishment.) For a while there your body seemed to be collaborating, but is now no longer a Mr. Nice Guy! Further weight loss becomes much more of a challenge, you have to severely restrict your calorie intake or vigorously exercise to rev up your metabolism. Keeping your weight under your body's setpoint will further require continuous vigilance and some level of deprivation.

It is important that you understand and accept the way your body works, and the difficulty involved in fighting its natural inclination. You will be more likely to lose weight if you realistically see the challenge you face. Losing weight and keeping it off is more difficult than climbing Mount Everest, because you are never comfortably at the top. A better analogy may be swimming upstream and barely staying in one place, and doing this *all the time*. We are not saying that you cannot do it. No doubt you have pursued other difficult goals in your life. Most likely you have decided that, difficult as it was, these goals were important enough to pursue and attain.

In the course of your dieting, you will find that some days or weeks it will be much more difficult to stick to your diet. This is unavoidable, and your best recourse is to stop horrifying yourself over these setbacks, and to keep accepting yourself despite your not having a will of iron. Just keep doing your best until you get back on track.

You will also find that even when you stick to your diet religiously, your weight loss will fluctuate, sometimes a great deal, from week to week. The scale may even register a gain, when you have adhered to your diet perfectly. This happens because of water retention, and because of fluctuations in your body's metabolic functioning. You will do well to accept these fluctuations as par for the course, and concentrate on monitoring your eating. In the long run you will lose weight.

Popular wisdom suggests that weight slowly taken off is more likely to stay off, but there is no research supporting this idea. Keeping it off depends only on your continued restraint in eating, on your level of activity, and on how your new weight relates to your body's comfort, that is, your setpoint. It is true that very low calorie diets slow down your metabolism. This means that your body becomes overly efficient in metabolizing food, so that you must restrict your eating even more to maintain your weight loss. However, this effect is temporary, and your metabolism returns to its normal level two to three weeks after you discontinue the diet. The advantage of quick weight loss is that it is quick; you see results right away, which encourages you to stay on your diet. You have to deprive yourself more, but for a shorter period of time, and you get to be thin sooner.

Another popular idea is that weight loss on liquid

diets quickly returns, because the weight was not lost "naturally," and the dieter did not learn to eat in a "normal" fashion. We and the researchers in the field disagree with this notion as well. True, it is not natural, or not usual to forgo solid food for weeks or months. But it is also not natural to eat one slice of toast and coffee with artificial sweetener and skim milk for breakfast, one apple for a mid-morning snack, lettuce with lemon juice and vinegar dressing and four ounces of low-fat cottage cheese for lunch, and so on. Either way, severe restraint of your "natural" hunger is necessary for weight loss. After reaching your goal weight, further "unnatural" restraint will be necessary to maintain it. The advantage of liquid diets is that you are more likely to stick to them; your choices are severely limited, so that you are not constantly tempted to indulge in more than the three to four ounces of whatever foods may be allowable on your non-liquid diet.

After reaching your goal weight, you will indeed need to know calorie contents of various foods and learn different eating habits, so that you can maintain your weight. You can prepare for this while on a liquid or semi-liquid diet, or when you get off it. The fallacy here is that fat people are fat because they have poor eating habits, and they must be taught proper ones in order to be thin. The evidence suggests that fat people's eating habits are no worse on the average than thin people's. In order to be thin, they must adopt better eating habits. But most dieters are intelligent enough to comprehend the issues involved. If they are to become and stay thin, they must learn to think and choose rationally among available choices, be it while on a liquid or solid food diet or on a maintenance plan.

THE CASE OF RHONDA

Rhonda agreed with most of her friends and relatives that her weighing thirty-five pounds "too much" resulted from her diet and poor eating habits. But when she went to a series of weight reduction seminars at the Institute for Rational Emotive Therapy in New York, she realized that she and almost all her close female relatives had fairly high setpoints and that even fairly good eating habits would practically never keep her or them ideally thin. So she stopped damning her "poor habits" and herself, even when she was able to lose only fifteen of the thirty-five pounds she would have liked to lose, and then, keeping to her regular eating habits, she was able to maintain her new weight, which she now began to see as "fine."

In the following chapters we give you tools for weight loss. These will be mostly psychological tools, that is, ways of thinking rationally which will maximize your chances of achieving your goal. We believe that there is no one ideal diet that you should follow. Your learning how to make clear and rational choices concerning your eating, and your not having self- defeating demands about yourself and your dieting experience are the most important tools to success. We will spend some time discussing general psychological well-being, and ways of handling everyday life hassles, because how you handle every other aspect of your life affects your stress level and your success with dieting as well.

Notes for Chapter 7.

1. Groves & Rebec, 1988.
2. Pasquali, Besteghi, Casimirri & Melchionda, 1990.
3. Mathus Vliegen, Tytgat & Veldhuyzen Offermans, 1990.
4. Harris & Martin, 1989.
5. Briddon, Beck & Tisdale, 1991.
6. Nachman, 1959.
7. Mayer, 1968.
8. Woods, Figlewicz Lattemann, Schwartz & Porte Jr., 1990.
9. Castro, Vieira, Chacra, et al., 1990.
10. Morley, 1989.

11. Klyde & Hirsch, 1979.
12. Faust, Johnson, Stern & Hirsch, 1978.
13. Sclafani, 1984.
14. Faust, Johnson & Hirsch, 1980.
15. Blundell, 1990
16. Schneider, Monahan & Hirsch, 1979.
17. Hays, 1991.
18. Beck, 1990.
19. Sanacora, Kershaw, Finkelstein & White, 1990.
20. Stanley, Kyrkouli, Lampert & Leibowitz, 1986.
21. Cooper, Bloom & Roth, 1986.
22. Ono, Kawamura, Shimizu & Ito, 1990.
23. Gardier, Trouvin, Orosco, et al., 1989.
24. Saland, Wallace, Reyes, et al., 1987.
25. Cooper, Bloom & Roth, 1986.
26. Grossman, 1984.
27. Marcus, Wing, Ewing & Kern, 1990.
28. Leander, 1987.
29. Levine, Enas, Thompson, et al., 1990.
30. Wurtman, 1988.
31. Wurtman, 1987.
32. Facchinetti, Giovannini, Barletta & Petiaglia, 1986.
33. Giugliano, Cozzolino, Torella, Lefebvre, Franchimont & D'Onofrio, 1991.
34. Giovannini, Ciucci, Cassetta, Cugini & Facchinetti, 1991.
35. Scavo, Barletta, Vagiri, Burla, Fontana & Lazzari, 1990.
36. Kraft & Vetter, 1991.
37. Wolkowitz, Doran, Cohen & Cohen, 1988.
38. Robert, Orosco, Rouch & Jacquot, 1989.
39. Wilber, 1991.

8

Philosophical Changes For Weight Control

Your emotional states, as well as your "good" and "bad" eating actions, largely stem from your thinking about yourself, about other people, and about the world. Through the years, you have developed ways of perceiving and evaluating different situations, including some implicit ideas that you may have never fully examined. Your way of looking at the world, your philosophy of life, can make the difference between constructive and self-defeating patterns of behavior, between healthy emotional states and severe distress. Rational-emotive therapy (RET) focuses in on your main irrationalities. It helps you re-examine your irrational philosophies and replace them with more rational and self-helping ones. How well or badly you react to different situations can be explained through the following ABC model of RET:

"A" is the Activating Event: usually negative events or situations, or thoughts about bad things that may occur in your life. An example of an "A" is the observation, "My boss expects that I work overtime without extra compensation," or "I have failed an exam," or "I was rejected by a person I want to love me," or "I am overweight."

"B" is your Belief about the adverse situation. You have both rational and irrational Beliefs about events. The rational Beliefs are realistic evaluations of the situation and a wish or a preference that it not exist. A rational Belief about your demanding boss can be: "This is quite an inconvenience and it would be good to find a way of rectifying the situation." A rational Belief about the observation, "I am overweight," would be: "It is sad and unfortunate that I haven't been able to lose weight thus far. I wish I would improve my life by losing some." Thinking rationally is often different from "positive thinking," in that it is a realistic assessment of the situation, with a view towards rectifying the problem if possible. It would not be rational to be happy about being overweight, or about having to deprive oneself of food in order to lose weight.

Irrational Beliefs fall into four main categories: (a) demandingness or *must*urbation, (b) awfulizing, (c) low frustration tolerance, and (d) self-downing.

Demandingness is an absolutistic judgment concerning how oneself, others and the world all *should* be different than they are:

"I should have been able to lose the weight already!"

"My family must be more supportive in my attempts to lose weight!"

"The world owes me respect and appreciation and ought to give it to me whether or not I lose weight!"

"My life must be free of stress, for then and only then could I lose weight."

"I shouldn't have to work so hard at controlling my weight. Life must not be this unfair!"

All these demands would be rational if they were preferential rather than absolutistic—if you would realize that many situations indeed are not fair or ideal, but still take responsibility for your own actions in spite of this fact. Accepting reality and taking responsibility is the first step towards behavior change and successful dieting.

When "awfulizing," you lose sight of the real significance of an undesirable situation (e.g. being overweight) and blow it out of proportion to the point where nothing else matters. *Awful* tends to mean *totally* bad—or even *more* than bad, which of course nothing could be!

> "It is *awful* and *horrible* that I am overweight. I can never enjoy my life, never be happy *at all* unless I am thin."

> "It is *terrible* that I have to keep dieting and denying myself foods I love, in order to look thin!"

As long as you maintain that it is *awful* not to be thin, or *terrible* to work at being thin, you will make happiness be indeed elusive, and you will make dieting more difficult than it need be. Realistically speaking, being overweight does not make anyone's life one hundred percent bad. There are in fact many sources of enjoyment other than having a thin body, if you will only acknowledge and take advantage of them.

Low frustration tolerance (LFT) is the belief that one cannot stand discomfort or frustration—for example the discomfort of exercise, hunger, or deprivation of pleasant tasting food:

> "My life is full of stress and I can't say 'no' to food when I'm under stress. I *must* not be deprived under such conditions!"

> "I just can't get myself to wake up earlier in the morning to exercise. It's too hard!"

> "I just couldn't resist that chocolate cake at the party! I *must* have it when it tastes so good!"

"It is too hard to say 'no' when friends or relatives are urging me to eat!"

These "I can't" statements really mean that you *won't* put in the effort necessary to lose weight. Once you decide that losing weight is a more important goal than the goal of avoiding stress, hunger pangs, or fatigue, there is no reason why you would not be able to lose it. With a gun held at your head you could stay away from the chocolate cake, because the consequences are clear-cut. As long as you remain conscious of the consequences of eating or not eating the cake, the choice is clear and dieting is do-able.

"Self-downing" often results from your demands on yourself:

"I should have been able to lose weight. Since I haven't done so, I am a worthless piece of . . . "

"I have no self-control and I am a contemptible nothing that nobody could ever love."

Self-downers rate themselves as humans on the basis of their behaviors, usually focusing in on their less-than-perfect behaviors. Contrary to what you may have read in countless books on self-esteem, the key to happiness is not to convince yourself of being full of wonderful qualities. In reality, we all have positive and negative traits and tendencies. As long as you persist in feeling good about yourself only when you perform well, you are setting yourself up for self-hatred. Instead, as RET stresses, work at accepting yourself as a fallible human being, fallible but never subhuman, never unacceptable.

By all means strive to improve your life and rejoice when you succeed, but when you fail you can make yourself feel only sad and disappointed, not because this suggests or proves that you may be worthless, but only because you did not obtain your goal. Self-downing also leads to negative predictions about your future success. If you judge yourself as "unable to lose weight" as opposed to "someone who has not thus far been able to lose weight," the chances are that your pessimistic view will become a self-fulfilling prophecy.

At point "C" in the ABC model are the Consequences of your thinking, both behavioral and emotional. Irrational Beliefs often lead to undesirable Consequences:

> When you demand that life *should* be stress-free and that others *must* support you in your endeavors, you will then tend to be angry and bitter, and will refuse to take the responsibility of monitoring your eating as long as the goddamned world is not cooperating!
>
> When you think that it is *awful* to have to deny yourself food, you will be less likely to restrict your eating.
>
> When you think that it is an awful fate to be fat in a society that is prejudiced against fat people, you will most likely be depressed and less able to help change your weight.
>
> When you decide that it is too hard to resist temptation, you will not resist it. (Eating is always a decision, nobody forces your hand to pick up food and put it into your mouth.)
>
> When you see yourself as worthless because you are overweight, you will be unhappy, will lack confidence in your abilities to change your fate, and as a consequence will not likely succeed.

Rational Beliefs lead to desirable Consequences:

> When you decide that it is unpleasant to restrict food intake but that there are many other pleasures in life, you will concentrate on these other pleasures, largely stick to your diet, and tend to lose weight.

When you think that being fat in a society that is prejudiced against fat people is definitely a disadvantage but that you can live with it, you will be less desperate to lose weight, less emotionally upset, and more likely to succeed in reducing.

When you decide to accept yourself regardless of your weight, you will be less desperate and you will more easily make the effort needed to lose weight, in order to improve your health, social life, etc.

Every human being holds some rational as well as some irrational Beliefs. RET shows you how to be emotionally undisturbed and to behave beneficially, by disputing your damaging irrational Beliefs and coming to fully believe your rational ones.

Stop Demanding that Life Should Be Easy or Fair or Any Way that It Isn't!

"It is unfair that I have to work harder than others at keeping my weight down. It shouldn't be this way!"

"People should always be nice to each other!"

"Sales people should not be so pushy!"

"I shouldn't have car trouble!"

"Innocent babies should not die of AIDS!"

"People shouldn't be prejudiced against fat people, or handicapped people, or anyone!"

"There shouldn't be natural disasters!"

"I should be able to enjoy all the foods I love as much as I want to!"

These statements are all reasonable, in a sense. They indicate how you might *like* the world to be. It is good and healthy to have *preferences*, and admirable if you try to change the world so that people are nicer to each other, cars run better, diseases are curable, natural disasters can be forestalled or avoided, and everyone can easily control their weight. But that word "should" is a tricky one. You can strongly prefer something without getting yourself upset, but as soon as you start demanding that, at all costs, things *must* be a certain way, you are being irrational and putting yourself on the road to much needless emotional distress. When you absolutistically demand something, you are no longer accepting reality. Yes, a rotten apple should fall from the tree straight to the ground and, indeed, it does. That is the way our world is set up. Babies should be conceived by a sperm entering an ovum. The sun should indeed shine brighter than the moon, the moon should be full once a month. Things should be as they are, at least for now. Irrational demands are always about things being different than they are. But empirically, things that are not a certain way, don't have to be that way, or else they would be. You may be able to get them to your liking, but there is no guarantee, and no reason why you *must* definitely be able to.

"Self-control is too hard. It *shouldn't* be this hard."

"I deserve to have it easier. I deserve to give up overeating with no effort."

"I *should* be able to get away with overeating. Other people may suffer ill effects, but I *shouldn't* have to."

A famous Hindu guru was once quoted as saying, "Life is a vessel of tears and never-ending misery." This is admittedly not a cheerful outlook but it does have the advantage that one will never be disappointed by life, and happily surprised at times. Life is indeed difficult, partly because of the real difficulties we must overcome in order to survive, and partly because of our own innate desire to always do better, to overcome new challenges, to self-actualize. Happiness is experienced largely in striving towards a goal, not in having attained things, because our nature is always to want to go on to the next endeavor.

Having the philosophy that life absolutely *should* be easier will only increase your misery. On top of the actual problem you encounter, you will have the added anger and low frustration tolerance brought on by your refusal to accept the situation for what it is, and just doing your best to change it or live with it.

Many people also have the demand that life *should* be fair, that misery *should* be equally distributed among mortals. (Of course, we'd accept a little extra happiness without worrying about fairness.) There are two logical problems with this proposition. First, there is no clear-cut way of measuring each person's misery. Different people, at different times in their lives and for different reasons, have difficulties. Different people react with different degrees of anguish to the same types of situations. How then do we come up with an exact equation of the amount of happiness and unhappiness that *should* be experienced by each of us?!

The second problem is that there is no particular reason why life should be fair. If fairness were an intrinsic quality of human existence, life would naturally be fair. Just as the laws of physics make the rotten apple fall from the tree, so the laws of nature would make everyone's life "fair." But from even a casual observation of "life," we find innumerable examples of unfairness. We can easily find plenty of examples of people who have had more adversity to deal with than we have, and people who appear to have had an easier life. On a very basic level, we see that everyone is born with a different set of characteristics: different physical appearances, talents, and intelligence. Humans come in infinite variety, and not all variations are equally valuable to ourselves and to those around us. From birth on, we start out in an "unfair" situation.

Most humans have a sense of right and wrong, and try to be relatively fair in their dealings with others. Even so, we dispute about the "right" and "fair" solution to countless dilemmas. Philosophers, clergy, lawyers, politicians, in fact, most humans in general spend a lot of time trying to figure how things ought to be. But the more rational of us realize that a fair society is not a given, it is only something to strive for and probably never quite reach.

Less rational persons, though confronted with stark examples of unfairness—such as babies born with the AIDS virus or natural disasters—stubbornly refuse to see reality, and persist in a belief in a just world. They want to believe that life is intrinsically fair (even if in some situations are obviously not), you reap what you sow, what goes around comes around . . . Such super optimists have a dire need for structure, for having meaning in life, for order in the Universe. Indeed, it would be unsettling to live in a world where we could not guess the consequences of our actions, where anything could happen (where apples fell *up* occasionally?!). We are therefore grateful for the laws of physics, which allow us at least to deal with the physical world in a fairly predictable way. Moreover, because we do want an orderly and just world, we have created societies and constructed rules which we decided would best provide fairness. This is a rational course of action for humans who value justice and equality. But if you believe, in spite of all evidence, that life is or should be naturally fair, comforting as this idea may seem at first glance, it leads to emotional disturbance. First, you may blame yourself for your misfortunes even when in reality you had nothing to do with creating them. You *must* have done something to deserve them, right? Physically handicapped people, people with chronic diseases, people with weight problems, they must all be bad people somehow. Second, your devout belief in a just world will lead to chronic anger. "If people do not act right, if life is not fair, it damn well *should* be! I will not accept this, and I am going to stay angry until things change!" . . . And anger usually does little to make the world a better place.

Putting yourself down and damning the world both lead to unhealthy emotions and to ineffective behavior. A better goal would be for you to see reality for what it is and to make the best of it.

It is not fair that you have to work harder than many others at losing weight, but so are many other things unfair. You can live with the unfairness. There is no one and no thing to be angry at. So you weren't lucky enough to have genes for thinness. But your being heavy, or having to work very hard at not being so, is not a deserved punishment for any of your other attributes. It is simply one of your traits, one that is not particularly to your liking. Further, there is no rational reason why you *should* have been able to lose weight by now. You are allowed to be a fallible human being. In fact, like it or not, that is what you are. So stop bemoaning your fate and putting yourself down! You have the choice of continuing to upset yourself about the unfairness of it all (and probably decrease your chances at successful dieting), or to accept your "lot" in life and make the best of it.

Conquer Low Frustration Tolerance!

"I *can't stand* frustration and pain. I *can't bear* being deprived."

"It is my nature to overeat, I can't help it."

"I *need* immediate gratification."

"Life is too boring without sweets, I *must* have them."

"If I don't eat, I'll feel anxious, and I *can't bear* feeling anxious."

"If I just think about stopping, I'll get so upset, I'll have to eat more!"

Do any of these sound familiar? They are just a sample of the type of thinking involved in low frustration tolerance, another form of irrational thinking and feeling where realistic preferences are turned into absolutistic needs and demands.

Most things worth having require some sacrifice, usually more than you expect. So much, in fact, that perhaps you would not set out to accomplish some goals if you could clearly foresee the extent to which you would have to inconvenience yourself to reach them. You would think, "I couldn't put up with that much grief and aggravation and frustration!" Indeed, many people tend to underestimate their own capacity to withstand frustration. Naturally the initial reaction to stress is to try to avoid it, but most of the time if you don't face the frustrating problem at hand you will have additional frustrations later. Naturally we often look for short-term comfort instead of long-term pleasure, and we look so hard that we convince ourselves that it is really our only choice, as it would be "too hard" to get the long-range goal.

If it were easy for you to keep your weight down— that is, if your body was naturally thinner—you wouldn't be reading this book. You may want to reach a weight that is at the lower end of your body's natural setpoint, or under your body's setpoint. If so, in the process of losing weight you will feel hunger and discomfort a significant part of the time. There is no way around this reality. When you do reach your goal weight, you will have to continue frustrating yourself by not eating everything your body craves. If your goal weight is well below your setpoint, you will most likely experience a low-grade level of hunger some part of the time, as your body will constantly be giving you signals that it "prefers" to be heavier. If your goal weight is at the lower end of your setpoint but not below it, you will have less of a problem with hunger pangs, weakness, or other physical signs of hunger. However, you will still have "mouth hunger" to contend with—

you will have to deny yourself tasty but fattening morsels of food that would bring your weight up to where you started. It is frustrating to go against your natural impulses for food, but it is not necessarily an unbearable state of affairs. It is simply a tradeoff between eating everything that you want and looking the way you prefer.

> "It is too hard to control my eating. I can't stand the discomfort of fighting my urge to eat."

> "I cannot do it. It is too hard."

These are untrue statements. When you attempt to control your food intake but fail to do so, you are really deciding that you do not want to forgo immediate satisfaction for the long-term benefits of weight loss. Hunger is unpleasant, but it is not so unpleasant that you must eat in response. More rational self-statements are as follows:

> "Being deprived of food is unpleasant, but I can tolerate the unpleasantness."

> "There is no reason why I should get what I want immediately; I don't have to eat whenever and whatever foods I want."

Your frustration from deciding to forgo delicious or plentiful food can be compounded by situational factors: people offering you food, people encouraging you to eat fattening foods.

> "I can't refuse when other people keep offering me food."

It certainly takes even more determination to stick to your diet under these circumstances, but it is still not impossible to say "No." Staying away from certain dishes does not have to be an insult to the hostess; there are other ways of showing appreciation for her efforts.

Contrary to many people's way of thinking, you are not responsible for other people's feelings. If the hostess at a party "becomes" upset by your refusal to have a slice of chocolate cake, she is in fact making herself upset. She can make herself see that you are only watching your calorie intake rather than trying to put down her baking skills. She has the irrational Belief that on such a special occasion you *should* go off your diet, and that if you only cared about her or about the event being celebrated, you would. So she is unnecessarily getting herself upset. If you care about her feelings, you might want to take her aside and explain your feelings and priorities to her. Or give her some RET! But you certainly don't need to undermine your goals in order to indulge her inappropriate upsetness.

> "When I am bored or lonely I need to eat. I cannot tolerate these feelings without food."

Unless you are approaching starvation, you never *need* to eat. (Even then, you only need to eat if you want to stay alive.) Further, eating is not likely to improve your mood beyond the time it takes to chew and swallow the food. There are many other activities which involve contact with others, learning new things, expanding one's horizons, which are better antidotes to boredom and loneliness.

> "Since my life is not going the way I want it to go, I must eat to make myself feel better."

Once again, eating will not make you feel better, except for the few moments it takes you to chew and swallow. But it will only frustrate your goal to lose weight. You can work harder at the real issues that are troubling you, and in the meanwhile you can stand being deprived.

"If there is a celebration I must eat to fully enjoy the day."

Why must you "fully enjoy the day?" A celebration is a time when there is something positive happening, so that the additional pleasure of food is even *less* required than usually. Of course, there are ways of structuring your diet to allow for one larger—not huge—meal, and this can be a rational, planned process; it does not have to be an act of losing control.

"I'm too old to change at this age; it's too hard to learn new habits now."

It may be a little unsettling to make changes now, but it is never too hard to learn new habits. It is still a matter of comparing what you have to gain by making changes, with what you have to lose by sticking to old habits.

You may have other excuses for why you cannot tolerate dieting. To control your eating, you'd better become aware of these excuses, and then strongly dispute them. See that you are indeed capable of working towards a goal you find worthwhile.

A tool to overcome low frustration tolerance is the hedonic calculus. You make a list of the positive and negative outcomes of different courses of action, give positive or negative numerical values to each outcome, and total the scores to find which outcome has a higher positive rating. Below is an example of a hedonic calculus concerning whether or not to restrict food intake, but each person will have their specific outcomes to consider.

Positive Outcomes	*Rating (1–10)*
Better health	_____
More energy	_____
More attractive to sex partners	_____

More career opportunities   _____
Fitting into a favorite outfit   _____
Wearing a bathing suit   _____
. . . What else can you think of?

_____

_____

Total   _____

Negative Outcomes

Hunger pangs   _____
Possible weakness   _____
Deprivation from food   _____
Nervousness and irritability   _____
Depression due to deprivation   _____
Moodiness   _____
Fatigue   _____
. . . What else is on your list?

_____

_____

Total   _____

On a scale from 1 to 10, how important are these and the other outcomes on your own list? If you add up all the scores for the "positive outcomes" and the "negative outcomes," which wins out? Are you overweight enough that dieting could lead to significant changes in your life? Or are these changes not worth the constant self-control you would have to exert in order to lose weight? You can more easily decide to stay away (or not) from certain foods, if you are clear about the consequences of your actions.

Stop Awfulizing!

"It is *terrible* and *awful* that I don't have a thin and attractive body that would draw sex and love partners to me."

"It is *awful* to diet and to change my eating habits."

"It is *awful* that I have to work harder than others at losing weight."

"It is *horrible* that things are unfair—my body type, age, metabolism."

When you awfulize, you concentrate on a negative reality in your life and blow it out of proportion: "This is so bad that everything else fades by comparison; I cannot possibly enjoy any of the other aspects of my life until this one problem is solved." But in fact you are choosing to give so much importance to that one problem. You could instead choose to be displeased about it, keeping in mind other things in life that are pleasing.

Another aspect of awfulizing is blowing out of proportion the negative consequences of a problem: "I am fat and ugly and no man will ever want me." Reality is that while it is generally more desirable in this society to be thin, other positive aspects of a person do compensate for one imperfection. Further, people's tastes vary a great deal. For example, there are men with a clear preference for large women, and it is just a matter of making the effort to meet them. A woman who thinks that she is too fat to be attractive may actually be too thin for the tastes of some men!

"It is awful that some people may make fun of my weight, or may assume that I am less smart or competent than thin persons."

Indeed, this is an undesirable state of affairs, having to work extra hard at convincing people of your intelligence and talents. Reality is such that some of us have to overcome prejudice and narrow mindedness, because of our weight, height, color, ethnic background, or customs. You can choose to be outraged about this, to rage at people who cruelly stereotype you, or you can wither away in despair, giving up hope of anything good ever happening to you. But these are over-reactions, going far beyond the extent to which the problem affects your well-being. When you define something as *awful*, you are in effect saying that the situation is more than one hundred percent bad, that nothing is worthy of enjoyment as long as this problem persists. With such a viewpoint, you are likely to suffer all sorts of emotional turmoil, including anger, depression, and anxiety.

It is very human to over-react and exaggerate the magnitude of a problem, but it is not in your best interest to do so. You can believe a situation is unfair and calls for change, but rationally you'd better accept that it is not awful. It just is another hurdle in your path. Once you see that very few things are truly awful, you will stop feeling sorry for yourself, and take responsibility for dealing with your predicament: handling bigoted people, and handling your body's strong tendency to stay at that high weight that you dislike.

It is not awful to be deprived of what you want to eat, not horrible to change your eating habits. It is only un-pleasant. There are other pleasurable activities that you can substitute for the pleasure of eating. Most importantly however, remind yourself that losing weight is hard, *as it should be*. Just about nothing is *awful* (one hundred per-cent bad or *more than* bad), especially not this reality in your life.

Accept Yourself!

"Since I've failed at losing weight, it proves that I'm a loser who deserves to suffer."

"A fat slob like me doesn't deserve love or respect from anyone."

"As long as I look as I do, I don't deserve to enjoy life!"

"Being overweight makes me worthless, sub-human."

You wouldn't want your friends to reject you based on one flaw, when there are so many other things you have to offer! But that is exactly what you do to yourself when you feel bad about "yourself" for being overweight. A person some feet away might only be able to know you as your outward shape, but even he would guess that there is a whole person inside that body. And you are certainly in a better position than an outsider to know that your weight is just one of your many attributes. So why would you feel bad about *yourself* just because you feel bad about your weight?

The self is an illusory concept to start with, because it is the sum total of your past and present behaviors, thoughts, attitudes, beliefs, experiences, feelings and sensations, as well as your future potential in all of these areas. Because it involves such a large number of attributes (from the color of your eyes to your talent in table tennis, to the size of your feet to your taste in art . . .), and because you cannot foresee your future, you cannot accurately and completely evaluate your self. It is safe to say though, that if you've made mistakes in the past, you will likely make mistakes again; if you were less than perfect in the past you will continue to be imperfect.

So what? Where is it written that you, unlike other mortals, must at all costs be perfect or even close to it? If you had to be, you would be by now. What we are suggesting here is a reality check. It is only in your mind that you *have to* excel, at anything or everything. Of course, it would be very nice to excel at most things. Indeed, we recommend that you try and do your best. But realistically, you are entitled to do the bare minimum to get by. All your accomplishments are just a bonus, something to enjoy, not requirements. You don't *have to* do anything to prove that you are worthy of existing.

You are an acceptable human simply because you are a human. Just as all squirrels are acceptable as squirrels, all cats are cats by definition, you certainly qualify as a human. Whatever flaws you may have can never make you unacceptable or subhuman. As a full-fledged human, you always have the right to seek out pleasure and happiness in life, which is a much better goal than trying to pass some test that would make you acceptable to yourself. Just as you now may choose to harshly judge yourself at every turn, you can decide to choose self-acceptance, and work at making the best of what you have, so that you maximize your enjoyment of life.

Some people do not accept themselves because of a flaw they have, but others even go a step beyond and invent flaws, to prove to themselves that they are unacceptable. Frequently, people and especially women, decide that they are overweight when no one else would view them as such. It is impossible to exactly determine each individual's ideal weight. However, we do know what the average ideal weights are, for each sex, for different ages, and this leads us to interesting findings. Among "normal" weight college students, fifty-eight percent of females and twenty percent of males classified themselves as overweight.[1]

This phenomenon starts at a young age: Seligman and co-workers,[2] 1987 found that among five hundred children fifteen percent were overweight, but over half the girls labeled themselves as overweight. Thirty-one percent of ten-year-olds reported "feeling fat." It appears that children and young people easily make themselves insecure about their bodies. Any noticeable fat is seen as too much. In a study of body image, researchers asked female subjects to stretch their hands in front of them and estimate the width of their hips by the distance between their palms; most of them overestimated the size of their hips.

As a society, we have been indoctrinating ourselves that we *should* be thinner than we are. As human beings, many of us appear to have an innate tendency to put ourselves down, to find fault and magnify faults within ourselves. So, if being thin is important, those of us who have a tendency to denigrate ourselves, become convinced that we are larger than we should be, heavier, and definitely not up to par.

Were we to cure humanity of its obsession with thinness, it would still not be cured of obsessing and self-downing. If you are one of those persons who insist on not accepting yourself with your extra pounds, you would find other flaws to lament. There will never be a human being, including yourself, who acts and looks perfectly. It is a losing proposition to make feeling good about yourself contingent on good behavior and good looks.

Throughout our life, we exist in bodies with certain genetic tendencies which place certain limitations on our quest for perfection. These limitations are different for each individual, though within the population there is a normal or bell-shaped distribution of each characteristic. Few people are very tall or very short, and most are average. Few are geniuses or mentally retarded, and most are of average intelligence. Few are artistic geniuses, few are unable to draw a straight line, and most of us with some coaching can manage drawing simple pictures. Few have perfectly clear skin and few have severe acne, and most have some skin problems sometimes. Few are very obese or emaciated, most are average. The list goes on indefinitely. We prefer to be at a certain point along the spectrum of each of these characteristics. However, reality is such that most people will be average, few will have extremely positive or negative traits. You can only stray so much from the genetic tendencies with which you are born. To continuously rebel against your fate of having been born with your own and not others' genes is certainly irrational, overly-frustrating, and fruitless.

Your wanting to improve yourself and your situation in life is a positive characteristic. A rational reason for wanting to improve yourself is to improve your life conditions—for example, to get a job or a spouse, or to do pleasurable things. It is also rational to want to gain mastery over your world. But it is not rational to improve yourself in order to *like* yourself. A rational view would be the following: "Here I am, born with some positive and some negative tendencies. This is the material I have to work with, and I accept that reality (what else could I reasonably do?). I choose to accept myself, even like myself, with all my positive and negative tendencies. I allow myself to be a fallible human. Because I like myself and want to make myself a good life, I will work at overcoming negative tendencies and fully benefiting from good ones. If sometimes I fail, I will still accept and like myself, but I will look for new ways to overcome my difficulties."

The tendencies to judge yourself and to demand that you perform well at all times may be genetically encoded in human beings, because there is evidence that people in all societies and in all times have judged themselves based on their performance. (Perhaps we created a God to judge us out of our own wish to be judged.)

Evaluating your performance and always striving to improve it certainly has an adaptive purpose. Those who try harder do achieve more. Even more so in the time of our ancestors who hunted for their food, survival depended upon being very vigilant, lest one be killed by a hungry animal. In modern society this hyper-vigilance is no longer necessary, because our work in most cases does not involve life or death situations. The irrational belief that "I must do well at all times" is actually counterproductive, leads to poor emotional and physical health, and often sabotages actual accomplishment.

If you think you *absolutely must* do well, anxiety, guilt, and depression will follow those inevitable times when you make mistakes. You can also develop physical problems, such as ulcers from the constant self-induced stress of having to be perfect. Consequently, with these emotional and physical problems to contend with, your successful performance becomes less probable. Further, the belief "I must perform well" is likely to lead you to have a high level of arousal which does not help you perform most tasks. There is an optimal level of arousal for getting things done. Too little arousal or interest will lead to lowered performance, as will too much arousal, concern, and anxiety. Somewhere in between lies a healthy concern and interest in doing a good job which will help you perform to your best capacity.

We can hypothesize that if pre-historic cave people did judge themselves in terms of their performance, this may have been rational and adaptive. If they did not perform well, they died—that is, had no worth. But our lives are very different. Since with the industrial revolution most of us in Western society are no longer in any danger of starvation, it no longer makes sense to equate your worth as a person with your accomplishments in any particular arena.

How does one determine one's worth? There are two ways: worth to others and worth to self. Worth to others includes behaviors such as helping or pleasing others, and attributes such as height, weight, attractiveness. Worth to others does vary: some people have a larger number of behaviors and attributes which are easily pleasing to others, though different people often value the same person differently. Further, without changing yourself, you can seek out those to whom you can be of most value, thus maximizing your "worth to others." Most of us appreciate being appreciated, but many of us appreciate it too much, so that we don't feel that we are acceptable as humans unless we can please others a good part of the time. Most of us, in fact, do please others some portion of the time, but if we demand that we always be pleasing and appreciated in order to feel good about ourselves, we are certainly setting ourselves up for failure.

A more rational world view would be that it is good to please others, but we are not obligated to do so at all costs. Our worth to others may increase or decrease from time to time and change from "other" to "other," but this is not reasonable grounds for self-denigration. It is not written anywhere that we must at all times or even most of the time be useful to anyone else. It is also not possible to measure how our talents or presence may have in the past or may in the future influence others. So how do we decide when we have done enough? Not very easily!

Worth to yourself is "What can I do for me?" "How can I bring myself immediate pleasure *and* long term satisfaction?" This is a rational way of evaluating oneself, not for the purpose of self-judgment, but for practical planning. Not "What does it mean about me as a person that I am overweight?" (It means nothing!), but "How does being overweight affect my life? What are the pros and cons of trying to change this?"

Certainly you can get negative results from being overweight by our society's standards: prejudice, fewer social and career opportunities. Depending on the amount of extra weight, you may also have health problems. On the other hand, you can also get negative consequences from dieting: feelings of hunger, weakness, irritability, deprivation; the potential for gaining even more weight as a result of yo-yo dieting. If you are successful at keeping your weight down, for the rest of your life you will still have to fight your body's urges to return to a higher weight.

A rational decision concerning whether or not to diet and what goal weight to set would involve all these and other life factors. It would not involve the notion "I hate myself because I'm fat and I want to lose weight to like myself again." Such lack of self-acceptance is not only unfounded in reality (because you have scores of other traits and deeds that make up you, *yourself*), but is likely to lead to failure: "How could such a despicable loser as I ever succeed at sticking to a diet?" Not likely.

Thinking primarily in terms of "worth to self" is not a selfish view. It would be unethical and immoral to neglect the very person for whom you have primary responsibility—yourself. Further, unconditionally accepting yourself will allow you to make the best of the material you have to work with. Secondly, as a happy and self-accepting person you are likely better able to acquire "worth to others," because you will function better and be able to help others with your natural, learned and innate altruistic tendencies. Unconditional self-acceptance is a primary and almost essential tool in any weight loss plan.

The following are some ways of thinking so that you accept yourself regardless of your weight:

"Although I'd like to always maintain control around food, how well I maintain it is not a reflection of my worth as a person."

"I am a good person and can accept myself, even if I have lapses in following my food plan. There's more to me than my diet."

"I am more than just the pounds I weigh, more than just my body. I am a human being, not a lower animal. I can think and feel, and I can choose to be good to myself and to others in countless ways."

Find and Overcome those Irrational, Self-Defeating Beliefs!

If at this point you are skeptical of our approach, you may be saying "I'm not telling myself anything irrational, I just reach for the food without thinking anything!" We hold that most of the time you are indeed telling yourself quick "automatic thoughts" with which you give yourself permission to eat. But you may be right to some extent. Inappropriate snacking might have become a habit, that is, you've conditioned yourself to reach for certain foods automatically.

If that is the case, make yourself aware of your eating. The best way to do this is by keeping a log of everything you eat, if only for a week. If you do eat habitually, this will be an enlightening experience for you. We suggest only one week, because most people appear to be very resistant to this idea. For one thing, they think it is too much of a bother to carry a note pad around and stop to write in it each time they eat—one more instance of LFT! But their reluctance also stems from their reluctance to be faced with an honest list of *everything* they ate that day. For many of them it is too embarrassing, too disheartening.

If we analyze embarrassment, we find a lack of self-acceptance: "I am not acceptable to myself or others the way I am, with the way I've been eating. If people knew about my eating habits, they wouldn't respect me in the least. It's bad enough for *me* to see a list of food I ate today, but to show it to my counselor? . . . " Another irrationality is the "disheartening" part: "I can't face my true eating habits, they are too awful, and if I did face them, I would realize how far I am from eating as I "should," from eating so that I can lose weight.

Can you at this point dispute the above irrational Beliefs? How do possible poor eating habits, even gluttony, make you unacceptable as a person? Even if you are prone to bingeing, that is only one aspect of you that is not ideal (but not awful either) alongside your many other admirable qualities. Remember, you can't avoid being a fallible human, like everyone else. Further, your eating habits are changeable, regardless of how bad they may now be. Incidentally, you are probably blowing out of proportion the extent to which you differ from others in what and how much you eat; your eating habits are likely no worse than that of millions of other people. But even if you had the worst eating habits of all people in the whole world (somebody somewhere does hold that honor), you could accept that fact and accept yourself, as you set on the path towards improved eating. So, no, it wouldn't be awful to keep a log of what you eat, to be honest with yourself.

You will find that the act itself of writing down what you eat acts as a control. You will think twice before overeating, knowing that everything will be recorded. But at times when you still overeat, despite the log, *don't give up on the log*! Keep writing! This is just the beginning of your project. At this point, you are allowed to be quite fallible!

As soon as you become aware of what you are eating, you will be faced with the conscious choice of succumbing to or resisting appetite and habit. Whenever you do succumb, you are telling yourself certain self-defeating thoughts to allow your hand to grab that morsel and place it in your mouth (your hand does not have a mind of its own!). Before any of the edibles actually reach your mouth is the time to identify those thoughts and unmask their irrational nature. The best way to do this is by taking that same note pad where you've been faithfully logging your food intake and write down your crooked reasoning: "I am going to eat this because . . . It's too good to resist? . . . I deserve it after a hard day of work? . . . I shouldn't have to deprive myself so? . . . It's all hopeless anyway, I'll never lose weight?"

Once you have written down your irrational thought, ask yourself: "Where is the evidence that this statement is true and correct?" Answer that question. Fortunately, we can guarantee that you will not be able to find evidence to support your irrational thoughts. (That is why we call them irrational, or self-defeating.)

Next, ask yourself: How is it helping me to maintain this way of thinking that I have chosen for myself and which leads to such bad results? The answer here may be that it is only helping you in the short run—by giving you permission to enjoy your food. But it is not helping your life overall. Now that you have established that your way of thinking does *not* hold water *and* it is bad for you, you are on your way to change.

You may find that on a surface, "intellectual" level,

you become a rational thinker, but deeper down you are still rebelling. "No, I *must* have that ice cream!" "I *need* some sweets to relax me!" . . . or whatever your own version may be. To overcome this, dispute each "but" statement vigorously and consistently, each time you find yourself slipping back to your old way of thinking.

Old habits are hard to change, especially thoughts and beliefs that you have taken for granted most of your life, as if they were obvious and unquestionable. In order to uproot the irrationalities that you have devoutly (but often unconsciously) believed throughout the years, you will need to give your new rational way of thinking an equal chance. Be a scientist and examine your thoughts carefully. Identify those self-defeating beliefs, and see why they are untrue and worth replacing.

Now let us assume that you have followed our suggestions, you have stopped before eating, jotted down a few notes about the irrationality of your thinking, but you ate, stuffing the wrong food down your throat anyway! This can happen. That food item that you have made so appealing may have clouded your judgment. Or you hurried your disputing and never finished it properly. What do you say to yourself now? That you really have no self-control and are quite pitiable? Or that this disputing business doesn't work? Wrong on both counts. Expect set-backs and you won't give up the fight. You are allowed to screw up and we expect that you will. So don't beat yourself over the head about this, just go on with your day. Later, when you are not so hungry, look in your notebook and finish challenging your old thinking, find where it was faulty, and set your rational thoughts straight for your next encounter with FOOD.

After you've disputed your irrational thinking, you will come up with an Effective New Philosophy (E) that is rational, and that you can also use as a coping statement. A good idea is to come up with some coping statements that work for you, write them down, and say them to yourself whenever you tend to eat badly. For example, your coping statement might be "I *don't* have to have this muffin, I can *just* have the coffee with Sweet 'N' Low instead, and I will feel strong and in control!" or "I *can* deprive myself of harmful food; it's worth it." Instead of eating, I'll buy that tape I wanted, and I'll invite some people over to listen to it."

Notes for Chapter 8.

1. Klesges, 1983.
2. Seligman, Joseph, Donovan & Gosnell, 1987.

9

Practical Tips
for Weight Loss

This chapter will involve some practical suggestions about how and what to eat. We assume that most of our readers have a good knowledge of what constitutes a healthy diet. However, we included this chapter to make sure that you do not act on false information, and that you are not following some unnecessary restrictions that may have been suggested to you but which have no scientific support.

Though there appear to be such a variety of diets available for would-be weight losers, the effective diets have only two things in common: low-calorie and low-fat regimens. These two solutions are the bottom line. Below we present other factors for you to consider, but they are only suggestions, not absolutes to follow at all costs.

Counting Calories

There are no magic foods, and no magic food combinations that will miraculously "melt off" your body fat. Different foods have different numbers of calories, and the calories are composed of protein, complex and simple carbohydrates, and fat. To lose weight, you'd better, above all, restrict your calorie intake to a set amount. If you have more than twenty to thirty pounds to lose, a very low-calorie diet (VLCD) is recommended—that is, keeping your calorie intake under eight hundred calories per day. This will allow you to lose weight at a fast enough pace so that the results will keep you encouraged and on track throughout the dieting process.

Your metabolism slows down to some extent on VLCDs, and weight loss becomes more difficult as your body attempts to protect itself from starvation. Nevertheless, VLCDs are the preferred way to lose larger amounts of weight. Your metabolism will readjust to normal a few weeks after you increase your calorie intake.[1]

If you have less weight to lose, you could still choose a very low-calorie diet, but you might also decide on more calories per day, and slower weight loss. Starting with the number of calories you consume weekly to maintain your weight, for every 3,600 calories you save, you will lose a pound. So, depending on his average calorie intake, a tall man might easily lose two pounds per week at 1,500 calories a day.

Read labels, and don't eat foods if you are unsure of their caloric and fat content. Look at portion sizes, not just the calorie breakdown. Often the calories represent unreasonably small portions. For unlabeled foods, such as fruit, vegetable, meats or pizza, it is a good idea to buy a book listing the calorie content of common foods. After a while you will be able to guess the calorie content of most foods. (Make sure though, that you are honest and do not underestimate when you guess.)

Fat

Protein and carbohydrates have four calories per gram, but fat has nine calories per gram. This means that you must eat less food to keep your calorie count down if a high percentage of what you eat is composed of fat. For this reason, it is advisable to eat low-fat foods. Furthermore, even if you eat less and keep the calorie count constant, you will have a more difficult time losing weight if you keep fatty foods in your diet, because your body metabolizes fat differently from protein and carbohydrates. Research on animals, as well as data on humans shows that if, of the calories you consume, very few are fat calories, you will lose weight faster than if fat represents more calories in your diet.

One common misconception is that non-saturated fat is somehow acceptable for dieters. Whether the fat is saturated or not may affect your cholesterol level, but it makes *no difference* to your weight. One gram of fat is one gram of fat, whether it is found in vegetable oil, butter or lard.

Protein

You do not need a great deal of protein per day for good nutrition. About fifty-five grams will suffice. Weight-reducing diets based almost exclusively on protein lead your body to quickly lose water, not fat, and this loss is temporary. However, it is a good idea if you are dieting to have a larger proportion of your food in the form of protein, because protein will give you a sense of satiety. This strategy works for many people, but if you find a diet that is not particularly high in protein but which you can follow, there is no reason why you should not try it.

Carbohydrates

Complex carbohydrates (bread, pasta, potatoes, rice) are more desirable than simple carbohydrates (sugar, fruits), because they are metabolized more slowly. They will keep you feeling full and energetic for longer periods of time, as opposed to the quick burst of energy followed by hunger and weakness that sugar causes in many people. However, your goal is to keep your calorie count down, and if you find that it is easier to do so by giving yourself occasional sweet treats (e.g., non-fat frozen yogurt), by all means do so. If you eat sugar at the end of a meal, you will not experience that "sugar high" and "low."

Fiber

A high-fiber diet has been linked with a lower incidence of heart disease and lower cholesterol levels.[2-5] In addition, fiber is helpful for dieters because it gives the feeling of satiety. Fruits, vegetables, and bran products contain fiber. For most people fiber helps avoid constipation, though for some it brings it on. Too much fiber will probably give you gas, so don't overdo it. See how much your body can take.

Water

If you eat a great deal of fiber, you will need extra water to help digest it. Water in general keeps your digestive system clean and functioning well. It also makes you feel full, so that it is a good idea to drink as much water as you can. You may find it helpful to drink water before each meal, to take the edge off your hunger. Again, see what works for you.

Salt

Generally salt makes your body retain water, though some people don't find this to be the case. If your body does respond to salt by gaining water, you can decide to eliminate or reduce your salt intake. You can use salt substitutes, or herbs and spices instead.

Caffeine

There is nothing wrong with caffeine, if it helps you function, or gives you an energy boost at times. Watch out for the weakness you may feel an hour or so after you've consumed a cup of coffee, at which time you may be tempted to make yourself feel better with food. Like sugar, coffee gives you a quick high, followed by lowered energy soon after. But if you drink a cup of coffee an hour before a meal, this may be a good way to substitute a low-calorie beverage (with skim milk and artificial sweetener) for a higher calorie snack.

Alcohol

Learn how many calories there are in beer, wine, hard liquor, and mixed drinks. You will find that most of these are high in calories. You can incorporate a glass of wine or beer in your diet without too much difficulty, but more alcohol will leave too little room for more nutritious food. Another risk of drinking alcohol is that when you are intoxicated it is easy to lose hold of your determination to keep your calorie count down, and you may find yourself not only drinking but eating more than you had planned. Decide for yourself whether or not you can safely incorporate alcohol into your diet.

Vitamins and Minerals

No special vitamins or enzymes have been shown to "melt off" body fat. However, it is a good idea to take a multi-vitamin while dieting, because it is not likely that you are getting all the vitamins and minerals that you need from your restricted food intake. The multi-vitamin keeps your body functioning well, and keeps you from feeling sluggish or weak due to insufficient vitamins in your system.

How to Eat

If you eat many small meals a day rather than one big one, you will spend less time being very hungry and feeling low in energy.[6,7] Animal and human studies also show that you will lose somewhat more weight if you take in your calories a little at a time, rather than all in one sitting. However, you may find that you still prefer to just have one meal a day, and if this is how *you* can best stick to your calorie schedule, this is how you should do it.

It takes about twenty minutes for satiety signals to travel from your stomach to your brain. This means that if you eat fast, you will still be hungry even if you ate a great deal, until your brain receives the "news" about what you ate. You can choose to eat fast, stick to the caloric intake that you set for yourself, but expect to be hungry for a few minutes after you finish eating. Instead, you can learn to eat slower, or take a break in the middle of your meal (for example, make a phone call, or clean up around the house) so that when you finish the meal you no longer feel hungry.

Many of the popular diets restrict the types of foods you can eat, and result in weight loss because those few foods that you are allowed lose their appeal if continuously eaten. This is a good approach for many people, although the concept of "forbidden foods" arises—foods we can't have and therefore want even more. If you can keep within your allotted number of calories by including a slice of pie every day in your diet, you may successfully lose weight. There is nothing very wrong with any foods, except that high calorie foods such as pie take up a great chunk of the calories you can have for that day, and leave you hungry later.

You may find it a good idea to restrict your intake to a few foods that you like, so that you don't allow yourself to become overly tempted by a variety of tastes and textures. Some people find it helpful to stick to blander tasting foods, again so that they avoid temptation.

You may find it helpful to only eat one meal consisting of solid food each day, and take in the remainder of your calorie allotment in the form of protein drinks, spaced out throughout the day.

Exercise

Exercise can be classified as aerobic and non-aerobic. Aerobic exercise—jogging, cycling, swimming, walking— if done vigorously at least four times a week for at least half an hour each time, increases your metabolic rate and allows you to eat more without gaining weight, or lose weight without eating less. Non-aerobic exercise—weight lifting, muscle-building exercises—has little effect on your metabolic rate, but it increases your muscle weight. Muscle takes up less space than fat, and requires more calories to maintain. With muscle taking the place of fat you can look better without actually losing weight.

Exercise, especially aerobic exercise, is helpful in controlling your weight. If, over and above controlling your food intake, you are able to also exercise, this will certainly speed up your weight loss. However, if you want to lose a significant amount of weight in a small period of time, it is more important to make calorie counting a priority. Half an hour of swimming might burn off 130 calories and slightly raise your metabolic rate throughout the day. But these gains can be easily offset by five minutes of cake-eating, at around four hundred calories a slice. Exercising is healthy, increases longevity, and is a good way of maintaining your weight at a desirable level. For most people, however, it is not the solution for major weight loss.

Diet Aids

If you have a hard time getting started on a dietary regimen, diet aids can be a good idea. They give you the momentum that you need to get started. The most effective diet aid at the time of this writing is fluoxetine, a drug which is an antidepressant, but also helps with weight loss.

Food as a Positive and Negative Reinforcer

As we discussed earlier, the research in the field clearly shows that gluttony is not a main cause of fatness. Rather, people weigh what they weigh because that is approximately what their body's genetic coding dictates. There is a small group of overweight people with bingeing disorders, who do actually overeat, probably for psychological reasons. The majority of overweight people do not overeat, except insofar as everyone overeats in this society of plenty. Because food is a quick, easily-accessible, and very pleasurable pick-me-up, we all use it more than just to assuage our hunger.

In order to be successful at losing weight, try to understand your motives and patterns of eating. Do you overeat or does your body just metabolize food more efficiently? Do you eat mostly out of mouth hunger (because it tastes good), or out of stomach hunger (hunger pangs)? Aside from fulfilling certain physical needs, what function does food have for you? If you use food often as a pacifier, as a way of feeling better following unpleasant life events, or of filling up emotional emptiness in your life, make yourself aware of this.

There is nothing wrong with occasionally trying to make yourself feel better about life's hassles by doing something pleasurable, such as eating a snack even when you are not particularly hungry. But if you easily gain weight, you give yourself a second problem by eating to deal with your first problem. Adding weight gain to your original problem makes things much worse and creates a vicious circle.

Rather than only using food as an occasional reinforcer, some people use food as others use drugs, alcohol, cigarettes, or even video games—as an escape, a way of avoiding dealing with unpleasant situations. Even if you do not tend to gain weight easily, eating instead of working to solve your emotional and situational problems is destructive. Your unattended problems diminish the quality of your life. They do not go away, and may even become bigger and more difficult to solve as time goes on.

It is not surprising that almost all of us too often succumb to instant gratification. Like other organisms, we seek out pleasure and avoid pain; and we require much effort to use our human brains to gain control over our animal instincts. To help us go for instant gratification, a "pleasure center" has been developed. Researchers Olds and Milner hooked up rats' brains with electrodes and gave the rats a choice of pushing a lever which would deliver food to them or a lever which would deliver pleasurable brain stimulation. These rats starved themselves to death by continually choosing the pleasurable sensations over food. Food tasted all right, but the high they experienced through the electrodes was much more desirable.

The closest parallel to the rats' addiction to electric stimulation is, of course, drug addiction, under which humans do often forgo nutrition in favor of an immediate high. Eating is less intensely pleasurable than drugs (it is also less lethal, which makes it still a better choice) but it can still be used as a way of filling oneself with immediate stimulation and distracting oneself from a more unpleasant task at hand.

We humans have the same instincts for pursuing instant pleasure as do rodents, but we also have the brain capacity to assess the pleasures and discomforts our actions will bring, now and later, and to act in a way that maximizes long-range pleasure. A smarter rat would have thought, "If I stop occasionally to eat, I will live longer and thus get to enjoy longer these wonderful electric stimulations, therefore I'd better eat as well as stimulate myself."

Similarly, a smart human—you, we hope—assesses all the elements involved in maximizing short- and long-term enjoyment of life, and acts accordingly. For example, even when you are stressed out, you can choose to sit back and relax with a cup of tea for a few minutes before trying to fix the longer-term problems in your life.

Notes for Chapter 9.

1. Foster, Wadden, Feurer, et al., 1990.
2. Riccardi & Rivellese, 1991.
3. Arjmandi, Ahn, Nathani & Reeves, 1992.
4. Kohn & Ribeiro, 1991.
5. Anderson, Floore, Geil, O'Neal & Balm, 1991.
6. Jenkins, Ocana, Jenkins, et al., 1992.
7. Verboeket van de Venne & Westerterp, 1991.

10

Emotions and Eating

Food feels good—to almost everyone. And when you upset yourself over something it feels bad. What better solution than to offset your bad feelings with something that feels good? And what feels better than food? Of our two most reinforcing drives, hunger and sex, hunger provides the most prolonged and reliable pleasure. We are limited in the frequency and intensities of sexual activities, especially if we are males and are satiated and lose our erection immediately after orgasm. But food in Western society is almost always there, ready to console and soothe. Given its compelling delights, it makes sense that so many of us eat more when we are upset. Herein lies a paradox. Most of us know people who virtually stop eating when they are stressed or depressed. Others may eat more when upset but soon stop because the food quickly loses its hedonic or pleasure-giving properties.

Some research has found that obese people eat more to control negative emotions,[1-4] and this association between emotional eating and obesity increases with increases in body mass.[5] Research also shows that emotionally aroused obese people eat more when they cannot identify the cause of their arousal than when they could

173

put a label on what is bothering them. Non-obese people were not affected by failure to label their arousal.[6] Some research has also shown that although obese people are more emotionally responsive and more likely to engage in emotional eating than thin people, this only applies to snacks, not meals.[7] Overall, the evidence is quite strong that the more overweight people are the more likely they are to eat in response to negative emotions. But, ironically, this may result from their great desire to be thin. Because heavy people tend to be very conscious of their intake, many work at restraining their eating. But people who chronically deprive themselves may easily produce emotional stress by dieting and then give in to temptation when under this or other stress. Thus, people maintaining high levels of dietary restraint were asked to watch a frightening film.[8] People who maintained high restraint—*whether overweight or not*—ate more than people who were not under self-imposed dietary restrictions. This result was confirmed in a study of women of ordinary weight. The woman who actively worked on controlling their weight were more inclined to eat in response to negative emotions than were women who ate whatever they chose.[9]

That is, many dieters assuage their heartache by eating more. People on very-low-calorie diets have been shown to be able to maintain their regimen despite strong negative emotions during the first eight weeks.[10] After this, restricting their diet tends to make the dieter more sensitive to the emotional stimulus. One major factor that must be considered when examining the connection between emotions and dietary control is the effect of dieting itself. Like the many aberrant behaviors attributed to the obese temperament, emotional eating may be a result of the diet itself. That is, some researchers have found evidence that it is chronic or repeat dieting that creates the emotional sensitivity to dieting.[11,12] Nevertheless, if your goal is to lose weight, beware of your emotions.

Dieting and Depression

Many people who embark on weight loss programs are mildly depressed at the time. For this reason, we usually suggest that psychotherapy accompany, and sometimes precede, an attempt at weight loss. Depression can have endogenous roots—that is, the individual is physically predisposed to becoming depressed. It is called an exogenous or reactive depression when the individual does not have a history of depression, but a severe negative life event helps bring it on. In either case, however, depression involves irrational thoughts—about life in general or about certain events or conditions.

In rational-emotive therapy we use several methods to combat depression to help people work on losing weight. We show them how to find the irrational Beliefs leading to their depressed feelings, to dispute these beliefs, and replace them with a more adaptive new philosophy. In cases of severe depression, we often recommend anti-depressant medication to facilitate the therapeutic process.

Depressed overweight people are likely to focus in on the negative thoughts associated with their weight. These thoughts bring on their depressed feelings, as well as self-defeating behaviors that may keep them from reaching a more desirable weight. If you are experiencing severe depression, you may not be able to stick to a strict diet regimen, and failure may lead you to depress yourself more. So it is better to delay your dieting until you feel better in general and feel better about yourself, even at your present weight.

Unfortunately, even if you overcome your initial depression, and even if you were not depressed to start with, dieting itself can help bring on symptoms of depression. Deprived of food, your body slows down some of its processes, including the production of serotonin, which is associated with depression. You may experience nervousness and irritability, lack of energy, and weakness. These physiological changes make it easy for you to fall into a pessimistic, negativistic way of thinking. To keep your thinking and priorities straight, you will have to make an extra effort. We find that a support group with other dieters may prove very helpful.

THE CASE OF JENNIFER

Jennifer was often depressed and overate to distract herself and give herself *some* pleasure to counteract her depression. But then she depressed herself more about the overeating and her "fatness." She also noticed that when she did diet rigorously and got close to or a little below her setpoint, she felt more depressed. So she accepted this grim reality, used her RET to work harder to overcome her physiologically related depression, then used it to accept herself with her "fatness," and finally looked at what she was doing to make herself originally depressed—namely, "I *must* be a great writer and isn't it *awful* when I'm not and may never be!"

By using RET on these three levels of depression, Jennifer was able to make herself only slightly and occasionally depressed and to keep her weight reasonably down, even though she and several other members of her family seemed to be naturally on the chubby or fat side.

Dietary Restriction and Irrational Thinking

Anthony Sclafani [13,14] demonstrated that even rats will gain substantial amounts of weight if provided a "supermarket diet" consisting of a wide variety of high-fat, highly-caloric and appealing foods. He also found that rats that have genetic predispositions to obesity will gain far more on the same diets than other rats.

Animal research into obesity provides some fascinating insights into the role of diets for weight loss and gain. We can reasonably assume that rats and other animals do not overeat as a result of oedipal fixations, sublimation, or character weakness. If a rat gets fat on a diet, it is an effect of the diet and the rat's genetics and little else. Animals can be made obese with several methods, none of which involve learning, thinking or emotions.[15] Yet, without prescribed diets, calorie schedules and motivational literature, animals regulate their body fat levels with great precision.[16]

Diets themselves have been shown to produce the type of eating that is believed to cause obesity. Chronic food restriction often leads to bingeing.[17,18] As we will detail in the next chapter, most organisms have systems within their bodies that are set, and, that work to maintain a particular weight range. When you deviate from this weight, your body will encourage you to get back within the range. The greater the restriction on your eating the greater the forces your body will counter with to encourage overeating. A binge is one of the means your body may employ to bring itself into the nutritional balance it seeks.

Dieters usually classify foods as good and bad. This approach has been shown to often generate a result opposite from that which was intended. Dieters who classify foods as forbidden tend to abandon all restriction if they consume one of these foods. The "what the hell" effect is invoked and the dieter labels himself as a global failure. Since there is no point for someone who is a global failure to even try, the dieter continues to eat.

If you are a dieter you can do your own thought experiment about this. Think of the times you may have violated your own dietary plans. What happened? What were your thoughts about it? If you examine your thoughts you will probably find the basis for your behavior. Virtually anyone who has dieted has acted against her own plans and interests. In order, for example, to eat when you have set out not to, or to eat high-fat, high-calorie foods when you have planned to eat only low-fat, low-calorie foods, you must have done something to change your own thinking and point of view. Let's examine some of the beliefs that create the "what the hell" effect:

1) "If I eat at all *I am* a failure."

This absolutistic and overgeneralized belief tends to lead to excessive restriction and then to complete abandonment of control after the most minor violations of dieting. To say that you *are* a failure if you fail at any one particular task is the same as equating that task with the whole meaning of your existence. Can it be that your entire purpose in life is to lose weight? Obviously this is absurd. However, you may still only lightly accept this logic, end up attacking yourself for making even the most minor diet violations.

You can use this rational alternative: "If I eat too much it means nothing other than I temporarily failed at dieting. I can choose to refocus and ultimately succeed. But even if I never eat properly, I am still an acceptable human being."

2) "By going off my diet, it proves I *can't* stick to it."

If you endorse this belief you will also have other negative beliefs about your general efficacy. You start off dieting with grave doubts about your ability to accomplish any real change. You are almost *looking* for failure. Yet many studies have demonstrated that simply believing in one's ability to succeed will increase the likelihood of weight loss. [19,20]

You can use this rational alternative: "If I go off my diet it proves nothing more than I *choose* not to stick to it at that time. I can now freely choose to go back to it at any time."

3) "I *shouldn't* have to do this."

Ambivalence about a goal usually leads to irrational thinking. Many people feel compelled by others to lose weight, so they weakly adopt weight reduction as a goal. However, it is not something they are doing for themselves, and they commonly cannot detail too many benefits they will derive from losing weight. If you wish to succeed at any difficult goal, you must sincerely adopt it as your own. You'd better know why you want to achieve the goal. If not, each time you encounter hardship or some kind of barrier you will tend to retreat. It does not make sense to try to lose weight unless you deeply *desire* to do so. Otherwise your repeated failures will just "prove" that it's just *too* hard to lose it.

You can use this rational alternative: "I am heavy because of my biology and my actions, and I can choose to stay this way or change it. If I decide to change it, I will because *I want to*, therefore I *should* diet if I want to change."

4) "If go off my diet I will *never* be able to stop."

Several researchers have demonstrated that it is a common experience to feel out of control when breaking a dietary regimen. This is the time most binges occur. But all binges come to an end, and it is always possible to restart a diet. The belief that a violation [21] of your diet makes you a complete failure leads to two very negative effects. First, by making any deviation from your dietary program a "catastrophe" you will make yourself anxious. Second, you will put yourself (not just your behavior) down and encourage yourself to continue to violate your diet.

You can use this rational alternative: "If I go off my diet it will just be too bad! I'll do my damnest to get back on and figure out where I went wrong."

5)   "One *day* at a time."

Unfortunately, you can consume enough food in one hour to offset more than a day's (or sometimes a week's) worth of dieting. The one day at time logic can be perverted to a very self-destructive pattern of saying "I screwed up today, but tomorrow is another day." If you want to succeed at controlling your weight you'd better weigh every action independently. If you go off a dietary plan in the morning, the best thing to do is to make yourself go back on the plan that instant—*not tomorrow*!

You can use this rational alternative: "Every action I take is independent, and my body can store fat continuously. Therefore, days have little to do with my success. Rather, I will work continuously at succeeding without ever putting myself down when I goof."

6)   "The (situation, the people, the food, etc.) *made* me eat."

Others can effectively make your efforts at eating control more difficult. But they cannot control you or your actions. By giving up responsibility for your actions you will make yourself feel better for the moment. In the long run, however, you will teach yourself to believe in your own inability to regulate your own behavior.

You can use this rational alternative: "Others can tempt me or act to weaken me, but I am the only one that can control my actions. If I act contrary to my own goals, I will try to better understand my own actions and thinking, rather than blame others."

Assertiveness and Eating

It is difficult to be different from the average person. People distrust those that are not the same as themselves, and sometimes this distrust turns into dislike or hostility.

When your weight is the factor that makes you different, people are often hostile to you. Our society has determined that it is impolite to openly show disdain for one's skin color, religion, politics or other traits that may make one different. But this is not the case for fatness. The fatter you are the more likely people are to use your weight in a personal attack when they are angry or dissatisfied with you or with anything.

Over time a person who has come to be attacked, disliked, or scorned by others will often build her personality around placating others. It becomes very important to get people to like her. The thought of upsetting others tends to become highly unpleasant, even frightening. She therefore makes herself unassertive. She tends to keep her feelings of anger or resentment to herself. If she points out to someone that they are hurting, mistreating, or abusing her she fears that they will not like her anymore—or maybe even get angry at her! This commonly is the case of the very overweight person, who has concluded that in order to be accepted she must get others' approval. Unfortunately, unassertiveness doesn't work.

Think of the people you have known who are desperate to be liked. You will see that these people almost never achieve their goal. They may be tolerated or accepted but they are rarely liked by other adults on any kind of an equal footing. This kind of person is the class clown, the self-effacing "gofer," or the butt of everyone else's jokes. He or she unassertively yields to others' opinions or feelings. It is hard to be happy if you are this way.

On the other hand, you can be an assertive person. Being assertive *does not* mean attacking or ignoring others feelings. It means that you are willing to hold up for yourself fairly—*without* attacking others. We cannot stress enough the importance of this. A large number of people who deviate from dietary programs do so when they are ANGRY or OVERLY FRUSTRATED. The chart on the following page shows how this can happen:

Lack of Assertive Behavior and Diet

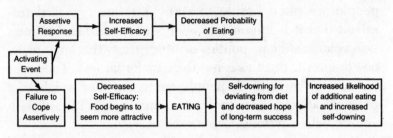

The scenario is common. Somebody impatiently infringes on your personal rights. This could be your boss, a co-worker, or a member of your family. Typically, they blame you for something that you did not do, or for something that was someone else's responsibility. You feel furious, you simmer for a while, but decide to let it go. After all, if you complain or assign responsibility to the right person someone might get angry, or they might stop liking you. So you don't "make waves." But you know this really solves nothing, because you are walking around angry and overly frustrated.

Your negative feelings that arise from your perception of your personal shortcomings often lead to negative thoughts about yourself. Or, as the preceding chart shows, to both increased self-downing and reduced self-efficacy. These feelings and behaviors make it very difficult to restrain your eating. After all, in order to suppress a force as strong as the desire to eat, you'd better feel good about yourself. Remember that if a person doesn't like herself, it becomes difficult for that person to make a sacrifice for herself. In the case of weight reduction, that sacrifice is the willingness to put off immediate gratification.

Since your self-downing leads to a reduction of your efficacy, you easily go back to overeating. Food first feels good, and gives short term fantasies of increased strength. For example, "Now that I feel good, I'll be able to take care of the people that hurt me; and I'll be able to stick to the diet tomorrow." But when tomorrow comes and nothing has changed, the eating leads to further reductions in self-efficacy and self-esteem. Another response is to blame the food or the situation, which externalizes control. That is, the person is saying, "The food controls me, I am powerless." Of course, this results in more eating.

Let's go back to the beginning. If the unassertive person had asserted herself instead of accepting the passive role of victim, she would have increased her self-efficacy. She would have felt increased personal strength and well-being, with a reduced likelihood of eating.

Afraid of Losing Weight?

Weight loss, or being fashionably thin, may not be desirable in some ways for some people. Some decide that the only way anything good could happen to them is if they lose weight. At the same time, they may feel that once they are thin, they will have no excuse for not accomplishing all they *should* accomplish. They are worried that they may not be able to handle intimacy or jobs that require a great deal of skill and responsibility. Within this scenario, the importance of weight takes on enormous proportions. "I must lose weight in order to be somebody. But I can't lose weight, for then I'll have to be somebody!"

Some insecure, self-downing people have the philosophy that their life would be wonderful if only they could become perfect, or close to it. (Conversely, they cannot enjoy life in an imperfect state.) The first problem they choose to work on is often the weight, since it so obviously exists. But once the extra weight is gone, won't there be other issues—insecurities in other areas, lack of assertiveness, problems in relating with people—to be dealt with? On some level these dieters are aware of a danger in losing weight and being faced with a host of other issues to deal with once they accomplish their goal. In particular, being thinner and more attractive to sex and love partners brings on new anxiety.

THE CASE OF MONICA

A thirty-year-old psychotherapy client related the following story about her past history. At twenty-four years of age, she weighed 155 pounds at five foot ten inches, and was constantly trying to lose weight. She had not been able to lose any significant amount for the previous few years, so she was starting to accept that she probably would not be able to. She was engaged to be married, while both she and her fiancé were in graduate school. Before the wedding, the two went on a trip to Europe, on which she lost five or six pounds. She describes the following: "When I came back, I was at my parents' house, and they have mirrors that make you look thinner. It turns out that their scale was also off, and when I went on it looked as if I had lost nine pounds. It was a strange experience. Instead of being happy about it, I panicked. I thought 'Now what? Now that I'm thin like I always wanted to be, should I still marry this man? Should I have different goals?' The panic subsided in a little while, when I figured out that I hadn't lost that much weight and I didn't look that different. I was still good old imperfect me, and my fiancé was still appropriate for me. I gained the six pounds back soon, and got married."

Of course Monica would have been imperfect even if she had lost a significant amount of weight. She was a thorough self-downer, had problems making friends, and felt that she did not fit in. Had she lost that little extra weight and "perfected" her body, her next step would have been to take a clearer look at her emotional and social shortcomings. She wrongly thought that it was more important to work on losing ten pounds than on improving her self-concept, and on the way she was relating to the world. She continued to struggle with her weight, but she actually gained another ten pounds slowly, by starving herself and then bingeing. With time, and later with psychotherapy, she worked on her emotional problems. She also learned to accept herself at 165 pounds, accept that she might never be thinner, but could still be a worthwhile and reasonably happy person. She continued to work at controlling her eating, though without desperation. With this new attitude and with some other changes in her life, she was finally able to lose twenty pounds. She found losing weight no longer scary, but neither was it exhilarating. She told herself that losing weight was nice but not necessary, and if she gained the weight back that would not be too bad, because her highest weight was not medically unsafe, and not terribly unappealing. At the end of the ten months for which the therapist was seeing her she had kept the weight off.

Monica was no more emotionally disturbed at twenty-four years of age than many of her peers. She was just someone who focused in on her weight as indicating all that was wrong with her world, and who saw thinness as the magical answer to everything. At thirty she was still far from perfect, but she developed more social skills, and, above all, learned to accept her imperfections as evidence that she was a fallible part of the human race like everyone else, rather than as evidence that she was a hopeless castout.

Being desperate does *not* help you to lose and maintain your loss. Desperation is also irrational, as it is quite possible to be unhappy though thin, as well as unhappy while fat. Seeing weight for just what it is, one aspect of you and your life, will allow you to feel less pressured to lose, and to be more rational in your thinking and planning towards your weight-related and other goals.

We don't believe that anxiety about losing weight or other emotional problems account for more than a small percentage of weight problems. There is no evidence that overweight people have more emotional problems than others. However, everyone does have some emotional problems, some difficulties in handling their lives. People who must use restraint to keep their weight at a desirable level are less likely to be able to regulate their eating when under stress, or when other psychological issues become intertwined with their dieting.

Notes for Chapter 10.

1. Blair, Lewis & Booth, 1990.
2. DuBois, Goodman & Conway, 1989.
3. Ganley, 1989.
4. Lowe & Fisher, 1983.
5. Van, 1985.
6. Slochower, 1976.
7. Lowe & Fisher, 1983.
8. Schotte, Cools & McNally, 1990.
9. Lowe & Maycock, 1988.
10. LaPorte, 1990.
11. Polivy, Herman & Warsh, 1978.
12. Polivy & Herman, 1976.
13. Sclafani & Springer, 1976.
14. Sclafani, 1989.
15. Fuller & Yen, 1987.
16. Harris Ruth & Martin Roy, 1984.
17. Herman & Polivy, 1984.
18. Greenberg & Harvey, 1987.
19. Edell, Edington, Herd & O'Brien, 1987.
20. Bernier & Avard, 1986.
21. Marlatt & Gordon, 1985.

11

Real Eating Disorders: Physical, Cultural and Cognitive Aspects

Perhaps the most irrational styles of eating are found in individuals afflicted with bulimia nervosa (BN), anorexia nervosa (AN) and the atypical eating disorders. We have shown in earlier chapters of this book that obesity is not associated with any psychological illness. This is not the case with eating disorders, which by definition represent a serious mental health problem. BN and AN are among the few psychological disorders that can be fatal.

There are many theories to explain the incidence of eating disorders, ranging from neurological to sociological reasons. However, the demand for thinness undoubtedly plays a role for many sufferers. Of course the desire to be thin will not in itself result in an eating disorder. As we have tried to make very clear, the compelling drive to be lean is widespread. So if this were the sole cause of real eating disorders, they would be almost universal. A person who suffers from an eating disorder will usually also have a personality disorder, although not necessarily a severe one.[1]

Certain characteristics of eating disorders make them unique among the psychological afflictions. First, girls and women are much more often afflicted than males.[2] The few men who are diagnosed with anorexia nervosa or bulimia nervosa tend to be unusual in some way. They are commonly gay or athletes, such as amateur wrestlers, in whom a small stature is prized. Second, eating disorders are often associated with childhood sexual abuse. A third characteristic of these disorders that make them uniquely difficult to treat is that many aspects of eating disorders are ego syntonic. That is, many anorectics and bulimics get reinforced by their disorder. Many profess dismay at the idea of the illness, but have also developed a powerful affinity for their extreme thinness or for the emotional release that purging brings.

The basis for making a clear distinction between obesity and real eating disorders becomes clear when we examine the two main disorders.

Anorexia Nervosa

The sufferer of this eating disorder characteristically exhibits extreme weight loss resulting from an exaggerated fear of gaining weight. According to the Diagnostic Manual of the American Psychiatric Association, the anorectic refuses to maintain a minimal body weight, falling to a weight fifteen percent or more beneath the minimum weight for her height. She expresses an intense fear of becoming fat, and perceives herself as fat in spite of objective evidence to the contrary. If she is a sexually mature female, she has missed three consecutive menstrual cycles as a result of her severe dieting.

In most cases the anorectic individual invests a great deal of emotional commitment to feeling hungry. Feelings of hunger commonly are strongly associated with the determination to be as thin as possible. This leads to feelings of depression and self-hatred after eating what would be considered by most to be a normal quantity of food.

The anorectic is typically quiet, passive, and withdrawn, a demeanor which belies her usual underlying disposition. She tends to be passive-aggressive, paranoid, depressed, and histrionic. Passive-aggressive styles are best shown by angry and overly frustrated individuals who mainly express their rage by sabotage. Anorectics tend to be very vigilant. They scan their environment for the potential violator of their small domain of control.

The anorectic often believes that she must please almost everyone; to be criticized risks the loss of essential approval. But the perpetual need for the approval leads to quiet rage and resentment. She is always vigilant for potential rejection and hurt. Her thinness is her means to comply with the "most" significant of society's standards, and to violate this canon, she thinks, is to flirt with rebuke. In fact, some researchers propose that the anorectic becomes "addicted" to her feelings of starvation. In one study anorectics were given naltrexone, a drug which is an antidote to narcotics. Naltrexone blocks the receptors in the brain to which opiates bind. Many anorectics who were given this drug began to eat.[3] This provided evidence that the chronic hunger that is induced in anorexia nervosa results in the production of endorphins, creating a type of "starver's high." Of course this only partially explains the maintenance of the behavior, and does not explain its origin.

Causation of Anorexia

The theories regarding causation of anorexia vary widely, but there are some common factors. Several of these can be seen in the scales of the Eating Disorder Inventory (EDI) (page 218). Many anorectics resist growing up and becoming responsible adults. Hilda Bruch concluded that many women with this disorder keep themselves in a childlike and asexual state by remaining extremely thin.[4] Frequently menstruation is reduced or stopped completely. The fleshy, characteristically feminine body is seen as contaminated. Fat, even in the most negligible quantity is viewed as flagrant sexuality. If not sexual, the

fatter body is seen as excessively large. The expansiveness
of the normal female body is seen as presumptuously large
and dangerous. It seems safer to stay small and unassum-
ing. To be normal-sized would invite adult challenges and
potential criticisms. After all, who would make demands
on the thin, frail woman whose diminutive stature makes
her seem like a perpetual child?

In spite of continual and excessive self-denial, the
anorectic always feels fat. Some actually see themselves as
fat by distorting their own view of their body. Their irrational belief that they are fat will tend to alter their visual
experience. As cognitive researchers have demonstrated,
our perception of the world around us is filtered through
the distorting prejudices of our attitudes and beliefs. Memory and perception are constructive. We *create* what we
see by synthesizing the sensations from our sensory organs
with what is already stored in our brain. Thus, the anorectic who literally sees herself as fat most likely actually does
see a fatter body than the rest of us see while viewing
herself.

THE CASE OF GLORIA

Gloria was attractive and perhaps slightly "overweight" at 120 pounds, but everyone, including her
boyfriend Milton, found her to be "zoftig" and sexy.
But she absolutely couldn't stomach her round stomach so she ate practically nothing to get it flat, got
herself down to seventy pounds, and had to have an
intestinal operation to keep her from dying. Warned
by her physician that to survive, she had to go up to at
least ninety pounds, she refused to do so, because at
seventy pounds her stomach was still round!—as were
the stomachs of most people in her family. Only after
several months was her therapy group able to show
her that a flat stomach was hardly an absolute necessity, and that she could be a happy person with a
"fat" belly. She finally compromised by getting up to

ninety-five pounds, still hating her stomach, but being able to live with it.

Gloria's cousin, Melanie, had a flat stomach all right, but sizeable breasts, which she hated because they made her "too feminine and therefore an inferior person." She was determined to go down to seventy pounds and be "titless," but when she saw how Gloria almost killed herself by futilely striving for a flat stomach, she decided that being feminine wasn't too bad, and settled for 110 pounds and fairly sizeable breasts.

The fact that anorectic states can be experimentally induced using surgical procedures or drugs has led some to conclude that, in some cases, anorexia nervosa has a physical basis. Recall from chapter 3 that animals can be made obese or emaciated by placing lesions in their hypothalamus. Damage in the lateral hypothalamic region of the brain results in cessation of food intake. If the animal is strongly encouraged to eat highly palatable foods, it will avoid starvation, but will maintain a much lower body weight than normal.

This line of research demonstrates that the control of eating and the perception of food as pleasurable is a function of brain centers. If this is the case, it follows that some anorectics may very well have neurological deficits. Virtually all the possible environmental or developmental causes of anorexia nervosa are also found in the lives of people who do not develop this disorder. It follows then that there may well be some kind of predisposition to this syndrome; but whether it is to be found in the appetite centers of the brain remains to be seen.

Irrational Beliefs of Anorectics

Irrespective of the basis of this syndrome, treatment can be effectively centered around disputing the irrational Beliefs peculiar to anorexia nervosa:

1)   "I *must* be perfectly thin."

The anorectic tends to equate her entire worth as a
human being with her thinness. The imperative towards
thinness is not based on any objective, cultural or health
standards. It stands alone as an elusive and sacred goal.
She will never be satisfied because perfect thinness is a
symbol, it has no real value on its own. As the anorectic
becomes thinner, she approaches but never quite reaches
her goal. Also, for the anorectic, thinness is abstract, not
concrete, and we cannot reach, or be, an abstraction.

The rational alternative is for the anorectic woman to
see the fallacy of regarding thinness as an absolutely, rather than a relatively, preferred quality. In other words,
"Thinness may be desirable, but I am essentially the same
person heavy or thin. If I can stand being heavier, it will
actually be easier to control my weight."

2)   Body fat is dirty, vile, and ugly. The more I have
     of it, the worse I am."

The irrational Belief that fat is absolutely bad is not
limited to anorectics, and is widespread in Western society. But anorectic people tend to take it to an extreme. If
persons with this disorder can be led to the conclusion that
fat is a natural and crucial part of the human body, they can
then see that it is not horrible to have some in their body.

An anorectic can use this rational alternative: "I would
prefer to have as little fat as possible on my body, but I'd
better understand why I have this preference. Fat is not
significantly different from skin, blood, or nerve tissue,
and it is essential for my survival. Because I cannot live
without it, it is irrational for me to define it as *terrible* to
have on my body."

3)   "Being small keeps me safe. A larger body states
     that I am competing with other women."

The illusion that being small protects a woman from responsibility and social demands is quite common among anorectics. They frequently see their emaciation as supreme femininity. The thinner, the more feminine, and the more distant they see themselves from having to fulfill the social demands that are seen as masculine. Ultimately, this state of mind is based on profound fears of social interaction, and on an irrational belief in the horror of one's interpersonal incompetence. By being physically larger, the anorectic fears that others will see her as more challenging. To an extent this is true. Specifically, most people will not be overly demanding on a small emaciated woman. But the costs of this social strategy are far greater than the real benefits.

An anorectic can use this rational alternative: "I can choose to avoid those responsibilities that I do not wish to take on, but making myself frail and weak will actually create a greater burden for me. I will be handicapping myself."

4) "No one can make me eat. By starving myself, I'll punish those bastards who have made me miserable."

Many anorectics feel as though others have stolen their life choices away from them, and their food intake becomes their last stand. Self-deprivation will be the way they will assert personal control and dignity. Of course, this is illogical because excessive deprivation only hurts the anorectic herself. But sometimes the elation she feels from hunger clouds this reality. Thus, the anorectic becomes even more insistent on her regimen as others "impose" their values on her.

An anorectic can use this rational alternative: "The best revenge on others is my leading a good life. Rather than hurting myself, I will do my best to take charge of my life and enjoy it, even if others try to control me."

5) "People will love me if I am thin and frail."

Fear of maturity is a frequent aspect of anorexia. Anorectics fear that if they develop into sexually mature adults, demands will be made on them. They fear that they will not be able to accommodate these demands and will thereby be rejected by significant others. In a related vein, the anorectic who lets herself become sexually or physically mature fears that she will lose the pampering that is typically conferred on children. So thinness becomes an irrational means to be continually taken care of—a condition she believes she needs.

Anorectics can use this rational alternative: "I prefer to be loved but I don't need love to survive. I do need food to survive. As such, it is foolish to starve myself to be loved. In addition, I have no guarantee that being very thin will really get me more love. At best it will only get me a different kind of attention. Instead, I can choose to appear and act like an adult and seek the love and affection that adults receive in mature relationships. This will be both physically and emotionally more fulfilling."

6) "If I get larger others will make demands on me that I will not be able to stand."

This belief wrongly holds that larger and physically more competent people are assigned responsibilities that the anorectic is sure she will not be able to withstand, and that she will then be proven incompetent and worthless.

Anorectics can use this rational alternative: "I can do my best to please important people in my life, but I don't have to always succeed, and I can stand their disapproval. I *can* handle adult responsibilities and if I fail at some of them I can always choose to accept myself anyway."

7) "Being hungry means that I am strong, and it will make me feel good."

As noted earlier, chronic hunger strongly affects the endorphin system in the central nervous system, leading in some cases to a feeling of well being that some derive from starvation. Anorectics also often irrationally believe that self-denial is a means to spiritual and personal improvement, and that the more they starve the more worthwhile they become. Because suffragettes who said they would starve themselves to get the vote for women [5] and because hunger strikers of every political denomination sometimes use starvation to help their cause, it is not surprising that anorectics also utilize abstinence to sacrifice themselves for "political" reasons. But, of course, they only harm themselves.

Anorectics can use this rational alternative: "I can fight if I want for women's and human rights, or my own rights, but starving myself to do so won't work and will only harm me."

8) "Being hungry is my just retribution for my sins."

This, of course, is self-damning nonsense. People who self-down frequently create sins for themselves, and anorectics are quite good at self-downing. They start off with the belief that they are bad and evil and then develop support for their premise by arbitrarily defining things they have done as being wicked.

A rational alternative that anorectics can use instead is: "I have done some things that I am not proud of, but this does not make me a *bad person*. Rather than punishing myself for sins of the past, I can work on doing things better in the future, so that I can both improve myself and help others."

9) "If I eat at all I will never stop. So I must not eat."

This is all-or-nothing thinking, and it implies that the anorectic has *no* self-control. First, it is extremely unlikely that anyone has *no* control over their eating. But the loss feared by the anorectic sometimes is self-fulfilling. By keeping oneself chronically starved one increases the likelihood of bingeing manyfold. The anorectic fears both fatness and loss of control so she creates the strategy of starving herself to avoid the risk of losing control with food. But the chronic hunger makes controlling the food progressively more difficult. Combatting this notion involves re-defining food as a necessary and pleasant aspect of living, and believing that she can control her eating and use food in moderation.

An anorectic can use this rational alternative: "Perfect control is not possible, and what's more it is not necessary. I really can control my weight without starving myself. And since in the long run starvation will inevitably lead to a loss of control, it is in my interest to try to eat in a way that food does not become my enemy."

10)   "The thinner I become the more special I am."

In a sense, this is true. People who have an unusual appearance in any way (in height, weight, facial features, or skin color) are "special" in the sense that they get noticed easily. However, this attention is not always positive. If you are exceptionally thin, others may feel pity, sympathy, or protectiveness, but usually not respect. And many think little of you for being so crazy! The anorectic is often afraid to try to be special based on her true talents and capabilities, for fear she will fail. She also often has the irrational belief that she *must be special*, otherwise she is worthless.

An anorectic can use this rational alternative: "If I want to be special, I can try to do well in my career, my artistic endeavors, my interpersonal relationships, or some other way. But I don't *have to be* special to enjoy my life. The more effort I put into improving my ways, the better it will be, but I don't have to *prove* anything to anybody. If I fail at something, I can still always accept myself, and I can try again!"

The irrational Beliefs leading to anorexia nervosa importantly interact with one's individual personality and social situation. Each anorectic's unique mix of beliefs, personality, and social circumstance result in many styles of this disorder. The cases of Gloria and Doreen serve to illustrate that very different people can be diagnosed as anorectics.

THE CASE OF DOREEN

Doreen was hospitalized when her mother first called one of the authors to arrange outpatient care when she was released. Her mother explained that Doreen, seventeen years old and an A student, never seemed to have any notable problems. During the last year, however, she became more and more concerned about her weight, even though she was far from heavy. Her mother noted that her older sister was quite thin, but did not take to the starvation extremes that Doreen took to when she was hospitalized. Doreen was very laconic and seemed quite annoyed during her first session. Although tall and attractive, her exaggerated thinness made her seem very frail. This impression was accentuated by her soft and abrupt style of speaking. It was clear after talking with her for a few moments that she saw therapy as another unnecessary tribulation she had to painfully endure.

She denied having any problems or emotional difficulties and claimed she ate as much as she wanted. She insisted that she had never felt better. When asked why she thought others felt she had a problem, she indicated that her parents were the ones with problems and she was simply caught up in their disturbances. Her parents were immersed in an angry and contested divorce, and as a result she, her sister,

and her parents were undergoing court-ordered family counseling. She said all this was doing was increasing the rancor between her parents. They were separated and came together only for conflict. She calmly
mentioned that her father routinely made middle of
the night calls to accuse the mother of various impro-
prieties—usually of a sexual nature.

As difficult as it was to discuss any topic at all
with Doreen, when the therapy focused on her eating
habits her resistance increased. After a great deal of
prodding, Doreen told of her one "eating day." For
six days in each week she would limit herself to a
bland salad with no garnishes or dressing and a small
piece of fruit. On the seventh day she would allow
herself to "eat everything I want." However, her
reports of what she ate on the "eating day" clearly
showed severe self-restriction. When informed that
this style of eating was unhealthy, she angrily responded that her sister did the same thing, and the
only difference was that her mother didn't pressure
her sister. In fact, both her mother and sister were
very thin, and both indicated that they felt it was
important to watch their weights. Clearly, Doreen
was getting double messages.

Over the course of therapy Doreen began to
express tremendous emotional confusion about her
parents' separation. She had come to believe that she
had to protect her mother from her father's abusive
behavior. Yet she expressed immense discomfort at
being angry at her father. In fact, with time, she made
it clear that anger was her emotional theme. She was
enraged at her classmates for a list of betrayals, which
all seemed quite trivial. Exacerbating her anger were
intense feelings of suspiciousness—almost bordering
on paranoia. She would not allow herself to trust any
of her small number of friends. Her social life was
unusually limited for a seventeen-year-old girl. Unfor-

tunately, this lack of trust also applied to her therapist. She persistently maintained a cool and aloof posture that she rarely softened.

Doreen's refusal to participate in therapy led to a worsening of her condition, and she was eventually re-hospitalized. When the therapist followed up, her mother revealed that she was much improved. It seemed that as long as she was in the conflicted family environment she stopped eating, and she made her obsession with self-denial worse. At the hospital, away from the conflict, she improved.

Anorectics like Doreen tend to withdraw into their illness. Their self-denial becomes their strength and protection. For Doreen the pain of starvation, was less painful than the emotional pain she felt. Her hunger became a focus, a type of distraction that gave her purpose and control. Like many anorectics she would go into frequent remissions, but would suffer relapses whenever under emotional stress.

Bulimia Nervosa

A bulimic is an individual who has binges, which are periods of rapid, high-volume eating that are difficult to control. To offset the binges the bulimic engages in one or more of several maladaptive strategies to control her weight. The most common of these is purging or vomiting after the binge. The others are intense exercise or the use of laxatives. Thus, for a person to be diagnosed with bulimia nervosa he must binge on a regular basis and also employ a maladaptive strategy to keep from gaining weight. Like the anorectic, the sufferer of bulimia nervosa strives to be thin. But unlike the anorectic, who by definition is very thin, the bulimic can be at virtually any weight. Sadly, it is not uncommon to encounter a bulimic who is quite obese. The irony of constant purging to become thin while staying or becoming fat is obviously cruel. Yet, as we will show, it is not that surprising.

Typically, the bulimic will follow a binge by forcing herself to vomit out the food that she just ate. However, because not all people who binge follow it with induced vomiting, the term bulimia nervosa has been adopted to describe the syndrome in which afflicted people repeatedly binge on huge quantities of food and then force themselves to purge. Bulimia nervosa (BN) represents a severe eating disorder. This is especially true if the afflicted individual experiences herself as being out of control, if she lives in fear of the next episode of bingeing, or if the bingeing and purging is creating health problems. BN, unlike obesity, has several well-researched causes. The sufferer is frequently, though hardly always, a victim of childhood abuse, or similar trauma early in her life.[6,7]

Biological Bases

Several researchers have proposed biological explanations of bulimia. One of these suggests that it is a disorder of appetite regulation. Recall that in chapter 7 we pointed out that the neurochemical peptide Y will generate bingeing behavior if injected into the brain. Because this peptide is ordinarily found in the brain, some people may produce a greater amount than others. In a comprehensive review of this matter in the *American Journal of Psychiatry* the authors found that there is often a genetic basis for the syndrome. They studied identical twins and fraternal twins and concluded that probably fifty percent of people with bulimia nervosa have a genetic inclination.[8]

However, one distinguishing characteristic that separates bulimics from anorectics is anger and instability. The bulimic tends to have a passive-aggressive style, reflecting a belief that others have done her irreparable harm and they must be punished. This belief goes with her feelings of thorough ineffectiveness as a person. Her purging and compulsive exercising can be sometimes viewed as an extreme reaction to her discomfort or rage.

The high frequency of borderline personality traits among people suffering from bulimia supports this view.[9-11] The bulimic behaviors can be seen as a special case of the self-damaging acts commonly performed by those with borderline personalities. Bulimics have been shown to be afflicted with some specific thinking distortions.[12] Whatever the psychological origin of purging, over time it may also take on a biological aspect. Some researchers have discovered that the feelings of satiety that normally follow a meal of carbohydrates tend to be interpreted by the bulimic as nausea. If the bulimics are given a placebo meal they do not feel nauseated. They only feel nauseated if given actual carbohydrates.[13] Therefore, the bulimics sometimes have an acquired feedback mechanism that provokes nausea when they consume carbohydrates.

Bingeing by itself, however, is not necessarily a problem. It may simply be a style of eating. Polivy and her co-workers have repeatedly demonstrated that bingeing is a universal consequence of eating restriction. Stay hungry long enough and you often will binge. From the point of view of self-preservation, bingeing is probably quite adaptive.

THE CASE OF CATHY

Cathy's first visit to one of the authors was for treatment for her anxiety and phobias. She explained that she had quit her job because of severe anxiety attacks, dizzy spells and urinary incontinence when distressed. Cathy was twenty-eight years old, thin, and quite attractive. The author was surprised when Cathy revealed that she had once been fat. In fact she had lost more than eighty pounds and said she would never, under any conditions let herself get fat again. Her basic strategy to stay thin was to purge everytime she believed herself to have overeaten. Her description of her typical diet suggested that the amount she considered to be "overeating" was increasing with time. She also took massive amounts of laxatives. The effects of her regimen were apparent—she looked pale and gaunt.

During the latter portion of her first session she said she felt she should stop making herself sick. When queried as to what she meant by this, she disclosed that she forced herself to vomit almost daily. "It's a habit now. I usually can get sick without even trying," she said with a bland tone, conveying a lack of sincerity about really stopping. When asked how she would feel about really stopping the purging and trying a maintenance diet to control her weight, she replied that vomiting was the only way she could control her weight. A psychological assessment revealed that Cathy was extremely depressed, anxiety-ridden, paranoid, angry, and prone to magical thinking.

Over the next few sessions Cathy gradually disclosed that she had been repeatedly abused by her father. She first mentioned that he treated her badly, and, after several weeks the story expanded to a grotesque drama. Her father would play games with her that included fondling her genitals, and having her watch him shave his genitals, so that he would look like a little boy. A favorite fetish of his was to have her dress in her halloween costume and ring the door bell. He would "let her in, and play games." These abuses went on for approximately eight years, until Cathy was about thirteen years old. The dread of his sexual assaults had become unbearable. She told him if he touched her anymore she would tell her mother. Fortunately, he stopped at this point.

Cathy never showed any anger at this history. Instead she expressed intense guilt that "she let this happen." When the psychologist asked what she should have done to stop him, she expressed that it would have hurt her mother so she couldn't tell her, and she was afraid if she told anyone else she would end up getting in some kind of trouble. She expressed a fear that if she were to have said anything about her father's abuse "everybody would think I was bad."

Despite these disclosures, developing a rapport with Cathy was very difficult. Her anxiety tended to create extreme withdrawal. She never really seemed to be there with the psychologist. She would speak to the wall or to objects in the distance. Rarely would she focus on the psychologist. When the discussion turned to a topic that she found perilous she would literally run to the lavatory fearing loss of bowel or bladder control. The dread of loss of bodily control was the basis for a growing agorophobia, or, fear of being in public places. Visits to supermarkets and department stores were especially anxiety provoking. Cathy described an overwhelming and suffocating terror that occurred with increasing frequency when shopping. The last time it was particularly bad, she lost bladder control and fled the store while completing a purchase at the checkout counter. She said that she couldn't even bring herself to enter her place of employment. Each time she would have to go in to obtain disability or health insurance forms, she said she would panic and shake, ultimately asking her boyfriend to go in for her.

Cathy claimed to desire to go back to work, and to be proud of the position she had risen to. Her co-workers were all men, which she volunteered did not faze her at all. She also volunteered that her boss had taken to making sexual advances to her. When the psychologist pointed out that the acute symptoms which led her to go on disability leave had commenced just after her boss began the sexual proposals,

Cathy remained silent. She acknowledged that one reason that she wanted to be away from work was her fear of leaving her son alone. She had developed an obsessive fear that she could trust no one with the care of her son. This led to even more resistance to leaving her home, and served similarly to isolate her son.

In the course of treatment Cathy revealed that she was now being treated abusively by her husband. He was an alcoholic and could not be relied on for even the most basic responsibilities of a spouse. He would be away for days at a time, and he could rarely account for his salary, which Cathy believed he spent to court other women. One particularly damaging irrational belief that Cathy revealed was that this type of treatment was inevitable and there was no point in trying to change it. She learned to challenge this and was able to leave this man, and despite intense pressure from him and her own family, she divorced him and moved away.

Over the next several months Cathy began to develop an understanding of the many irrational beliefs that provoked her misery, such as her demands for guaranteed security for her son, her absolutistic judgments of significant people in her life—which alternated between seeing them as all good and all bad—and her magical conviction that she was going to be singled out by cosmic forces for doom. Sadly, seeing her beliefs did not serve to diminish her symptoms. She still purges and excessively fears obesity—especially when under emotional strain. But her ability to recognize and dispute the beliefs that exacerbate this tendency has markedly reduced her bulimic symptoms. When she encounters a stressful situation she still has occasional panic attacks. But after therapy she is able to function autonomously and is able to raise her son in a satisfactory way, despite these difficulties.

Cathy's history is fairly common for women with bulimia nervosa. Her eating disorder was more symptomatic than problematic. She suffered from a host of psychological difficulties and her view of the world was deeply distorted. Her quest to stay thin apparently gave her a sense of control and distance from the world, which she believed to have her worst interests at heart. Cathy differed from most bulimics, in that she had stopped bingeing, but would still purge after virtually any meal. The following case is similar to Cathy's in her psychological profile, but the woman, Sonia, has a different history and manifestation of her bulimia.

THE CASE OF SONIA

Sonia was referred to one of the authors by a school psychologist who was distressed by both her depressed mood and progressive loss of weight. At the time of her first visit she was fifteen years old and an honor student in an urban parochial high school. Sonia was accompanied by her mother, who spoke only Spanish. It was immediately apparent that Sonia did not wish to participate in psychotherapy. She sat hunched over, approximating a half-fetal position. Despite her medical report, indicating a height of five feet two inches and a weight of eighty-four pounds, she seemed more diminutive than starved. Her demeanor and style were that of a ten-year-old child. Her speech was a combination of a whisper and a whine, as though she were in constant discomfort. She informed the therapist that she felt tired all the time and had not menstruated in a year. Her medical report described a young woman in poor health. She

was severely anemic, she suffered from gastrointesti-
nal bleeding from her chronic vomiting, her parotid
glands were swollen, and both her thyroid and estro-
gen levels were abnormally low. Her pediatrician
indicated that all of these ailments were a direct result
of her bulimic behavior.

Sonia revealed a personality style that usually is
common with anti-social personality disorder. She
had very high levels of anti-social, passive-aggressive,
paranoid, and hysterical thinking. According to her
psychological tests she was angry, suspicious, and
alienated, while desperately seeking affection. These
results were in direct contrast to her gentle, passive
style. But over time, it became apparent they were
accurate.

Sonia's father was a hostile alcoholic, in poor
health, who was separated from her mother. She
detested being around him but felt obligated to visit
him because of his ailments. She felt frustrated by her
mother's restrictions and foreign lifestyle. Her brother and sister had both dropped out of school and were
drug users. Sonia complained that despite their self-
destructive lifestyles they would always get more approval from her mother than she did. In talking to
Sonia, one got the feeling that she felt like an alien to
her family. She felt very different from, and ashamed
of her parents and siblings. Despite, her alienation
from all those who could be close to her, she desperately wanted their love. Yet Sonia felt helpless in
getting the love and approval she "needed" so greatly.
Despite this, she seemed to do everything in her
power to sabotage all her relationships—including her
therapeutic one.

Her attendance for scheduled appointments was
erratic, and when she did attend she would wedge
herself into the chair and adopt a "pollyanna" attitude.
She would maintain a gentle smile and consistently

avoid discussing any feelings. When in group therapy, she would ignore any women in her age range, choosing instead to vie for the attentions of the older women and the psychologist. During private sessions she would usually criticize the other group members in subtle ways. After a while it became apparent that she labored with a great deal of damning beliefs about most other people. She saw everyone as a potential competitor or adversary. Therefore, her interpersonal style was based on two strategies, to coopt or to defeat. Of course, this had the effect of isolating her from any real relationships.

Over the next year of therapy Sonia showed some slight improvement but she continued to fight all the way. One could never predict when she would come in for her appointments. Usually it was during some kind of crisis. It remained extremely difficult for her to express exactly what was troubling her. During this time she made two attempts at suicide. Both times she consumed large amounts of pills that she found around the house. The first time she was hospitalized for three days and released. After the second attempt she was treated in an emergency room and released when the resident concluded it was an accident. Sonia would downplay the attempts, so that the therapist was given the distinct impression that the attempts were performed just to be irksome. Passive-aggressive behavior defined the way she related to the world. Her lateness, absences, inappropriate emotions, and her silence in the group, were all attempts at striking back at those she believed were trying, in some abstract way to hurt her.

Sonia eventually quit high school, and took a job in a convenience store. She would occasionally come in for a session, but in most cases it ended up being some type of manipulative effort to get a letter for work absence or for disability.

Sonia represents the anorectic who received so much secondary gain from her symptoms that she refused to make any real effort to change. Her condition had served her well over the years to protect her from a hostile environment.

THE CASE OF BILL

Prior to Bill's first session he made several calls to the receptionist of one the authors to make absolutely certain that the therapist would accept his insurance plan. He went as far as having the benefits administrator of his employer contact the author's office to clarify his psychotherapy benefits to further assure his coverage. Prior to the initial session he indicated that the reason he was seeking psychotherapy was for help with his drug and alcohol abuse.

When the therapist met Bill he gave the initial impression of strength, competence, and emotional health. This false impression, known as the halo effect, tends to occur when the client either closely adopts or strongly violates what he thinks are the social prejudices of the therapist. Bill worked hard at presenting a good image. His hair was carefully styled, his nails manicured and he wore a perfectly tailored and apparently expensive suit. He entered with a broad and friendly smile, offering a handshake and a friendly greeting. After a few moments it became clear why he was successful as a salesman.

Towards the end of the first session he mentioned that he would vomit to keep his weight down. His weight was always a matter of concern to him. He described being very fat as a youth, and said he hated the way he felt when he would gain weight. Over the next few sessions Bill disclosed that he had been sexually abused by his father. He stated that he felt it was important to spend time on this trauma since he

believed that it was fundamental to his problem. The
author pointed out that this abuse may very well play
a role in his difficulties but his current evaluation of
the event was more significant at this time in his life
than the event itself. The author explained to Bill that
the belief that his past somehow disables him would
result in it doing just that. And since we cannot
change the past the only thing we can really change is
the way he views it.

Over time Bill accepted that his current views
and beliefs were more important than his history.
Some of these beliefs included his demand that others
treat him specially, that his self-destructive behavior
was a result of his childhood, and that since he could
not trust anyone, they had no right to expect him to
be trustworthy. He began to actively challenge these
beliefs and to clearly see that he was responsible for
his own feelings. With this he stopped his bulimic
behaviors, stopped abusing drugs (having only one
minor relapse in eighteen months) and was able to
terminate therapy with a new outlook on life.

Irrational Beliefs

The cases of people with bulimia demonstrate that
there are both many commonalities and differences among
individuals with this disorder. What most bulimics have in
common are some irrational views about the world around
them that can only work to make the symptoms and subjective distress worse. Although not all bulimics have all of
the following beliefs, most have some of them, and many
have ones not included in this list. The most important
procedure in dealing with this illness is to assume that they
are there and to actively dispute them.

The irrational Beliefs of the bulimic are often similar
to those of the anorectic. Many are derived from the
suspicious and angry style so common to bulimic people.

1) "I *must* purge if I feel full."

Many people with bulimia acquire the belief that the
feeling of fullness represents impending obesity. They
describe feeling fat, ugly or disgusting when they reach a
state of satiety. There are some physical correlates of this
feeling. Chronic purging leads to delays in gastric motility,
frequently leaving food digesting very sluggishly in the
stomach.[14] Other research has shown that bulimics classi-
cally condition their vomit reflex to be far more responsive
than in typical people, leaving the bulimic feeling as
though they must purge.

However, even if the bulimic has a physical urge to
vomit, she never loses free will over her body. She can
choose to submit to the discomfort of not purging. If she
has a fear of obesity, or an unpleasant feeling of fullness
that leads to the desire to purge, it can be overcome.

Bulimics often use *emotional* reasoning: "If I *feel* I
must purge, it must be the right thing to do." However, in
the case of bulimia nervosa, the first step towards healing is
to recognize that your feelings and sensations have come to
be distorted and unhealthy. At this point you might use
your rational mind to overcome the irrational urge to
purge.

A purger can use this rational alternative: "I feel like
purging, but I cannot trust my feelings right now. Refusing
to purge will not make me fat, but will make me healthy,
as I learn to control my eating without it."

2) "The *only* way to feel better if I have been hurt by
others is to eat and then to vomit."

Rage about their frustrations is frequent among bulimic people. They believe that the world treats them
unfairly and feel helpless in getting what is *owed* them. So
they silently rage at all the people who are not treating
them as they *should*. They also have irrational Beliefs, "I

must be loved by significant others" and "I *cannot stand* rejection." They frequently have low self-acceptance and self-efficacy, stemming from the beliefs that they are total-ly dependent on others, or on food for feeling good.

Bulimics can use this rational alternative: "I don't absolutely *need* love and approval from anyone, and I *can stand* disapproval. Instead of eating, I can find constructive ways of improving my life, which will bring positive long-term results, rather than just the bittersweet pleasure of a binge."

3) "If I stop purging I will *inevitably* get very fat."

Many bulimics do have an underlying tendency to-wards obesity, and if they were to eat everything they want, whenever they wanted, they would get fat. But this certainly does not prove the inevitability. Bulimics *can* diet instead of bingeing and purging.

They can use this rational alternative: "It is not true that I have to get fat if I stop purging. I won't let this irrational fear rule me!"

4) "Others are always trying to hurt me, and I can't risk trusting any of them."

Part of the extreme sense of vulnerability that many bulimics feel is manifested in this lack of trust. Of course if one doesn't trust, there will be no opportunity to form supportive, loving relationships. So by *needing* absolute trust they get very little—and then only trust themselves to control their weight, and presumably win approval, by purging.

Bulimics can use this rational alternative: "Nobody is out to get me, though it is true that sometimes people do things that hurt me, willingly or not. Food is no substitute for human contact, so I'd better control my weight sensibly and keep trying to find people worthy of my trust."

5) "Being full makes me dirty and vulgar."

This idea echoes modern society's disdain for fat, and the horror of showing it to others. So any sensation which might be associated with weight gain is abhorred. Once again, the bulimic unrealistically exaggerates the meaning of her feelings.

Bulimics can use this rational alternative: "I may feel dirty and vulgar when I eat, but that does not mean that I am really that way. My irrational fears of fatness are playing tricks on me. Feeling full occasionally will not hurt me in any way."

6) "Keeping thin will keep men from bothering me."

Implied in this statement is the idea that "I cannot handle attention from men," and ultimately probably the idea that "I cannot handle the rejection that will no doubt ensue from involvement with men."

Bulimics can use this rational alternative: "Some men may reject me, whether I'm thin or overweight, but some will like and accept me. If I do my best to avoid any interactions with men, I am actually eliminating any chance for forming a good relationship. It is in my best interest to be open to social relationships, and I can stand rejection when it occurs."

7) "I must punish those who have hurt me."

The bulimic feels a lot of anger that she has trouble explaining to herself. When she does reflect on the meaning of it she concludes that it is due to the wrongs of those in her past. One must examine the utility of hurting others close to them. There is a grain of truth in the idea that one's family members might feel sad or even guilty if one develops an eating disorder or becomes emaciated. However, their pain is very little compared to the extent to which the bulimic is hurting herself. Even if a family member harms a bulimic, her anger stems from her irrational belief that this person *must* at all times favor her and *never* harm her.

Bulimics can use this rational alternative: "I am better off working at becoming healthier and happier, rather than trying (perhaps unsuccessfully) to punish or evoke guilt in others."

8) "If I let my guard down, I will get hurt, and I couldn't stand that!"

People who suffer from bulimia nervosa frequently suffer from suspiciousness bordering on paranoia. They commonly have been hurt in the past and conclude that they will be hurt in the future. So they remain vigilant, always scanning for the next potential wound. All of us have a finite amount of cognitive capability, and if a major portion is spent on vigilance little is left for anything else.

The rational alternative: "I may have been hurt by significant people in my life, but this does not prove that others will hurt me in the future. Spending my energy anticipating that they will can only result in my being more alone and hurt."

9) "Purging is the only way they are going to comprehend my rage and disgust!"

Frustrated anger is a major etiology of bulimic behavior. Many bulimics make demands on all around them. They believe they have been denied and betrayed, and demand restitution. This is coupled with grave doubts in their own efficacy to obtain what is "due" them. So they silently rage at all their significant others, who are not giving them what they want. The others "should" know that they are hurt and angry. And others "should" make up for cheating and betraying them, and so on.

The rational alternative: "It would be very nice if everyone gave me what I need or want, but why *must* they? And how can anyone else know what I want, or how badly I want it? Why *should* they know?"

Rational-Emotive Treatment

Psychotherapy for the bulimic, like that recommended for the anorectic, differs from treatment for psychological problems because bulimia nervosa can be health threatening. Also, many of those afflicted insidiously find some of their symptoms desirable. Many of us have behaviors we would like to change but actually work at producing them. We do so because we want to eliminate a defeating trait, but do not *really* want to change it. For example, most drug abusers profess a desire to give up drugs, but despite all efforts they continue using them. Why? Because they crave the effects, the comfort and lifestyle, associated with their use. They really want to avoid the health and social consequences of using the drugs, but not the use itself. So they fool themselves by working against their alleged goals.

Bulimics typically follow a pattern. They may say "I want to change," or "I have to stop being this way." But they rarely mean that they are aspiring to stop the bingeing or the purging. Their binges are distracting and satisfying, their purges are protective and serve as a kind of physical catharsis. What they really mean is, "I don't want the hassles and consequences of my behavior any more— but I want to be able to keep doing it." The rational-emotive therapist works on helping bulimics understand that their anger and frustration is not due to their past. Instead, it is a result of the demands that they are making on the world, and those close to them. In therapy, the bulimic is helped to see that his judgments about others' hostility and danger may be distorted, and even if they are accurate it can be accepted with reciprocal hostility.

Compulsive Eating and Bingeing

An eating disorder that is not yet included in the current categories of the Diagnostic Manual is compulsive eating. Currently, there is research underway to develop new diagnostic criteria for binge eating disorder.[15] This diagnosis is for people who binge by eating a much larger quantity of food than is typically consumed and doing so in a relatively short period of time. In addition, they must have a history of bingeing at least twice a week for six months. The bingeing must result in the individual feeling out of control during the binge and having a sense of emotional distress after indulging in it.

We must look with caution at this diagnostic category. It is very common for people with weight problems to label themselves as eating disordered to help themselves comprehend their own misery with their weight. But as we made clear in the section on hunger the control of eating is an exquisitely complex process that is usually self-regulating. Most people are really just following physiological commands when they seek food and eat. There are of course exceptions.

Some people may eat an ordinary quantity of calories over a time period, while consuming their food in several intense episodes. For others bingeing may represent a distinct disorder. Parry-Jones and Parry-Jones in an historical review of bulimia present several cases of individuals who engage in massive and indiscriminate binges without ever becoming obese. None of these people were reported to purge or excessively exercise. They would gorge on animal entrails, many pounds of organ meats, or entire small animals. The fact that women who suffer from the tendency to eat compulsively tend to have male alcoholic relatives [16] suggests that this disorder may partially have a genetic origin.

THE CASE OF JOHN

John had been doing well in a weight loss group for some time, having lost almost sixty pounds before he began private treatment. He began bingeing, feeling out of control, and asked for individual psycho-therapy. John was thirty-seven years old when he began therapy and superficially appeared to be the kind of man who was always happy-go-lucky. Yet he was quite large. Six feet two inches tall and over four hundred pounds before he began the weight group.

In individual treatment John disclosed a misery that he hid from the other members of the group. His father was an alcoholic and so were two of his broth-ers. His mother was manic-depressive. Both parents chose to abuse him verbally and physically. He blamed his severe alcoholism on this history, which began in his mid-teens. John described himself as a "mean drunk" who was very much like his father. He told of his father's cruelty when intoxicated, which according to John was incessant. The only way his father would interact with him was with beatings, intimidation, and, worst of all, with ongoing ridicule. With his emotional pain obvious in his face, he told of the time he finally hit his father back—he felt both liberation and agonizing guilt.

Despite his rage at his father he used this event as evidence of his own worthlessness. In fact, John could come up with very few examples of anything positive about himself. He was extraordinarily self-downing. His own low estimation of himself led to his severe chronic anxiety. He was terrified of doing anything important on his own. In fact, dependency was a dominant feature of his personality. So when confronted with any life crisis he would lapse into panic or hypochondriacal dread. He was a familiar figure in most of the emergency rooms in his area, where he would regularly admit himself for chest pains, shortness of breath, or other life-threatening symptoms. Usually, he would be given a tranquilizer and sent home.

In therapy he learned the connection between his emotions and his bingeing. Self-acceptance became the theme of John's treatment so that he could live without dreading shame or rejection. After nine months of RET, John learned to stop self-downing and with that his anxiety and panic ceased. Despite the fact that he leveled at 370 pounds, he began to enjoy life.

Obesity and Eating Disorders

The behavioral problems that are classified as eating disorders differ from obesity in several respects. First, obesity is a physical condition that is not recognized as a mental disorder. The Eating Disorders Inventory (EDI) is a psychological test used to diagnose people with eating disorders. But it was not developed as an instrument to study obese individuals.[17] Nor have researchers been able to demonstrate that obesity is a psychopathological state or is a character disorder. However, in a study that utilized the EDI with those obese individuals who are similar to those with eating disorders, it was noted that these fat people do perform more poorly than others in weight loss programs. People battling obesity confront many of the same stresses as those with eating disorders. Both the obese and eating disordered individuals practice dietary restraint, both have strong negative feelings about their bodies, and both tend to experience many failures related to their eating. While the obese person has to fight against his own genetic tendencies, the anorectic or bulimic bat-

Table 1   Mean Eating Disorder Inventory Scale Scores

EDI Scale		Obese[a]		Anorectic[b]		Bulimic[b]		Student[b]	
		M	SD	M	SD	M	SD	M	SD
Drive for Thinness	(DT)	8.2	5.1	13.8	6.1	14.9	5.5	5.1	5.5
Bulimia	(B)	5.3	5.1	8.1	6.3	10.9	5.6	1.7	3.1
Body Dissatisfaction	(BD)	20.4	6.2	15.5	7.8	16.7	8.0	9.7	8.1
Ineffectiveness	(I)	3.9	4.4	12.1	8.6	13.3	8.6	2.3	3.8
Perfectionism	(P)	5.4	4.4	8.6	5.3	9.1	5.4	6.4	4.3
Interpersonal Distrust	(ID)	3.6	3.5	6.4	4.9	6.6	5.0	2.4	3.0
Interoceptive Awareness	(IA)	5.4	6.2	11.7	7.0	12.2	7.0	2.3	3.6
Maturity Fears	(MF)	3.1	3.5	5.6	5.8	5.6	5.9	2.2	2.5

[a] Abrams[18]

[b] Garner & Olsted[17]

M = Mean score
SD = Standard Deviation

tles something quite different. The EDI was administered to a sample of eighteen morbidly obese females and it was found that only their Body Dissatisfaction scale was elevated. This is concordant with the EDI data presented in Table 1. The table reveals that obese people score much more closely to the control group of students than they do to the anorectics or bulimics. In fact the only scale that the obese group was substantially high on was Body Dissatisfaction. This scale was designed to elicit disapproving beliefs concerning one's own body. When the scale is high the beliefs are considerably irrational and pathological.

Because obese individuals with eating disorders do perform more poorly in weight loss programs [19-21] the diagnosis of eating pathology is important. We have made clear in previous chapters that most overweight people do not have any psychological problems not found in other populations. However, this does not mean that there are not many heavy people who *do* have such problems. There are overweight people who make themselves fat primarily because of their eating disorders. Such people may be compulsive eaters, or sufferers of unusual eating disorders. However we classify them, they have an unusually difficult time adhering to dietary programs. This observation may explain the tendency to presume that obesity is a type of eating disorder. That is, many of the obese people *who seek treatment* may be drawn from that minority who do have eating pathology. Since the presence of the eating disorder will have made their weight loss more difficult, such a person is far more likely to seek help.

Notes for Chapter 11.

1. Steiger, Liquornik, Chapman & Hussain, 1991.
2. Schotte & Stunkard, 1987.
3. Moore, Mills & Forster, 1981.
4. Bruch, 1978.
5. Schwartz, 1986.
6. McClelland, Mynors, Fahy & Treasure, 1991.
7. Miller, 1991.
8. Kendler, MacLean, Neale, Kessler, Heath & Eaves, 1991.
9. Yates, Bowers, Carney & Fulton, 1990.
10. Yates, Sieleni, Reich & Brass, 1989.
11. Derksen, 1990.
12. Dritschel, Williams & Cooper, 1991.
13. Turner, Foggo, Bennie & Carroll, 1991.
14. Mitchell & Pyle, 1988.
15. Wilson & Walsh, 1991.
16. Kasset, Gershon, Maxwell & Gurott, 1988.
17. Garner & Olmstead, 1984.
18. Abrams, 1991.
19. Keefe, Wyshograd & Weinberger, 1984.
20. Wilson, 1976.
21. Marcus, Wing & Hopkins, 1988.

12

Philosophical Changes
in Living or
Don't Eat to Solve Your
Problems, But Solve Them!

The same principles of rational thinking that we have applied to your eating-related behavior also apply to every other aspect of your life. If you learn to think rationally about life in general, you will feel less stressed out and be more able to apply yourself to the task of losing weight and other important issues.

Though you never have to eat simply because you feel stress, it is harder to work to reduce your weight when you have other pressing issues to attend to. You may eat no more than the average person but, having been "blessed" with a more efficient metabolism than most, you are overweight. By deciding to lose weight you in effect are deciding to set out on a course of self-deprivation. In order to be successful in this endeavor, it helps to have few other hassles in your life, and to have good psychological tools for handling the hassles you do encounter.

These elements in your life that may need fixing generally involve both real, practical problems (such as work, love, or health problems), and involve emotional problems, which result from the way you *evaluate* these practical situations. If you rationally assess and accept the effects of certain situations on your life, you are likely to have less extreme emotional reactions and to act in ways most likely to improve these situations.

RET follows the prayer of Reinhold Niebuhr, "God, give me the strength to change what I can change, the serenity to accept things I cannot change, and the wisdom to know the difference." We also add that if God is not there to give us these virtues, we can choose to gain strength and high frustration tolerance, serenity and non-awfulizing, and wisdom and non-demandingness by learning to think rationally.

Because food is and always will be an intrinsic part of your life, you can always easily use it to avoid dealing with your problems. Therefore, controlling your eating actually involves running your entire life reasonably well, so you do not too often overindulge in the urge to eat. Let us now look at some common life problems to which you may over-react and then drive yourself to overeat.

Loneliness

Loneliness is a state in which people often overeat. Humans are social beings: they cannot survive without the help of others. Especially in pre-historic times, it must have been important to be with people and have their approval. Left alone without one's tribe, a person's life was in danger of being taken by wild animals, or by starvation. Human beings do indeed benefit from affiliating with others, nurturing emotionally, communing sexually, and co-operating economically. Today people can be much more self-sufficient than in earlier times, but we still seem to have an instinctive aversion to being alone or to gaining disapproval by others. Normal feelings of loneliness are common. But feelings of depressive, self-hating loneliness are created when we make the evaluation that it is *awful* and *totally unbearable* to be alone. We make predictions that we'll *always* be alone. In other words, we awfulize. You can fight the feeling of disturbed loneliness by examining your irrational beliefs that help create this feeling. You can strongly convince yourself that though it may be *preferable* to have pleasant companionship, it may be *less* preferable to have lousy companionship. Being alone is not necessarily a *terrible* state. You can see it as somewhat uncomfortable, and even a neutral state, which you can nicely fill with activities of your choosing. You can have your most creative and fulfilling moments when you are by yourself, if you allow yourself the freedom to do so.

Often, you may decide that there must be something very wrong with you if you are alone: "If I am alone that means that nobody wants me and I am worthless." However, being alone may result from conditions beyond your control, *or* from a rejection by others. But rejection by another person does not determine your worth as a person. It only determines that this particular person does not find it worthwhile to spend time with you. Overgeneralizing about this leads to great loneliness and depression, to negative predictions about the future, ("*Nobody* will ever want me!") and to feeling very sorry for oneself.

You do not have to overeat simply because you are depressed about being alone. Food is a very short term solution to this and other emotional problems. It only works while your mouth is full. Right afterwards, you may feel bloated, weighed down, unattractive, worse than before. And more likely to be alone! So if you are at times alone, dispute your disturbed evaluations of this state, and make the most of your time, instead of self-defeatingly overeating.

THE CASE OF ARNOLD

Arnold only overate when he was alone—especially when he had no woman living with him. Why? Because eating gave him something to do. He often ate out and pretended that the other diners were friends of his. He felt like a bigger, more solid person when he was heavy, and he felt soothed while eating.

Unfortunately, Arnold's preoccupation with eating kept him unattractive and took away the time and energy that he could have spent looking for female or other companions. So he got lonelier. And ate more. And got still lonelier.

When Arnold's Rational Recovery group helped him see that being alone wasn't *horrible* and did not make him an *inferior person*, he stopped making himself feel like a worm. He was then able to allow himself to eat *after* he had made some real attempts to meet new people. He soon had a live-in companion—and more friends than he could find time to be with.

Social Anxiety

Because the world is full of people, there are very few times when you really have to be by yourself. Often, you choose to be by yourself rather than take the chance of meeting new people and perhaps not being welcomed with open arms. Shyness is a common trait, one that often involves the irrational Belief, "It would be unbearable to be rejected, so I'd better not approach anyone unless I am one hundred percent sure that they want me to." This is just *one* possible evaluation of being rejected. A more adaptive philosophy would be, "It would be unpleasant if this person rejects me, but it won't kill me. If I keep approaching people, in the end some will take to me and I will have more friends or lovers than I started out with—maybe more than I will be able to use! Therefore, I can only win by approaching others and trying to socialize with them."

The fear of rejection can make you tongue-tied. You may think, "I'm nervous and I'll probably say something stupid, so I'd better be quiet." Instead, by deciding that you can live with rejection, you will take more chances. So what if you sound stupid? You can *allow* yourself that

common behavior. Even if people laugh at you, you know
you're not really stupid, just nervous. Paradoxically, the
more you allow yourself to fail, the less fearful thoughts
will screw you up, the more your natural personality will
come through, and the better you will do socially.

If you are generally nervous and uncomfortable about
social encounters, adopting a rational way of thinking is not
a total cure. The other half of the treatment is immersing
yourself in the situation you fear and dealing with it. You
may have low frustration tolerance about this: "If I don't
feel comfortable talking to someone, I shouldn't do it."
Well, you should, if you ever want to get over the discomfort. By thinking rationally, you will become *less* nervous.
By repeatedly forcing yourself into uncomfortable social
situations, your discomfort will disappear.

The "easy way out" of avoiding people is not really
easy. It keeps you in an unfulfilled state, with little friend-
ship, emotional contact, sex, or opportunities for professional networking. When you make yourself socially anxious, so that you have little left in your life other than food,
it will indeed be difficult to resist overeating. By expanding
your horizons and taking chances with new people and
new situations, you will leave less time for overeating, and
have less of a compulsive interest in it.

Interpersonal Problems

Now that you've learned to meet new people and
form relationships, your real problems may just be starting. You must learn to get along with these people if you
are to keep them around. Sometimes you wonder whether
they're worth keeping around, but then you may go back
to the neediness you still haven't totally overcome, and
decide to keep them around for a while. Or you may want
to relate to others out of healthy desire, not unhealthy
neediness.

The number one reason why you may become upset

around others and turn them off is if you demand that they *should* act, think, and feel the way you deem appropriate. You try to change them, but most of the time those inconsiderate bastards fail to comply. The truth is, people are going to act, think, and feel the way *they* want, not the way *you'd* like them to. That is why it is best to choose friends and lovers who are similar to you and who pretty much want to do things your way.

If and when you choose to make yourself outraged about things not being done your way, you will only make yourself miserable, and unpleasant to be around. On the other hand, if you realize and calmly accept that you only have limited control over what your friends and lovers do, you will feel better, less angry. You will still be sad and disappointed, but not horrified. You will also be able to better put to use the little power you do have, to help other people come around to your way of thinking.

If you want people to change, you'd better give them good reason to do so. An incentive. Unfortunately, they will rarely make major changes in their lives just to please you, unless you make it worth their while. So your task is to find the most clever way of getting other people to change their thinking.

You may, however, never come up with enough of an incentive for some people. Then you have the choice of putting up with the situation, or getting as far away from the person as feasible. It is good to look at your life as a series of choices about who you associate with, what you study, where you work, where you vacation, and so on. Because no one and no situation is perfect, you can reasonably expect that the people you choose to be with and the situations you find yourself in will be lacking in some ways.

If a person or situation becomes overly annoying, it is in your best interest to work at finding a better substitute, and perhaps hold on to the old people until new ones come around. The world and other people do not owe you happiness; it is up to you to make the best of your life. It is irrational (self-defeating) for you to become either angry or depressed over others' imperfections. They *should* be the way they are, for now. It is also irrational for you to feel justified in overeating because you have personal problems. Major problems will divert your attention from your diet to some extent, and you can at such times accept failings in your self-control. But don't hold the nutty idea that because you have problems with people and your life is therefore difficult, you *cannot* or *should* not have to monitor your eating. If anything, those are the times you'd better monitor it more carefully!

Work Problems

Conflict with co-workers is more dangerous than with friends, because it can lead to losing your job and to financial difficulties. On the other hand, work relationships are not intimate and it is not necessary to agree on many issues, or even to like each other. Nevertheless, work difficulties can certainly take their toll, especially if you have unrealistic expectations of yourself and your co-workers. Below are some choice irrational Beliefs about oneself:

"I must be perfect, I must not make mistakes, I must work faster, not waste any time."

"I must be above all reproach. If I'm not perfect at my work, I am worthless!"

"Others should never find out that I'm imperfect! I'll never be able to keep a job if they do!"

"I need for everyone at work to approve of me!"

"I can't stand the discomfort of criticism!"

If I'm ridiculed, everyone will think I'm pitiful, and that is awful! No one at work must ridicule me!"

Just reading these can make you feel stressed! Stress is not actually in the situation, it is in our heads—the feeling that things *must* get done! Even if your boss is threatening to fire you, things do not *have* to get done. It is in your interest to try to do a good job in order to keep it, but if you don't, life does go on. But even with a reasonable boss, you might be stressing yourself out by setting overly high standards for yourself.

There is no good reason why you have to be great, as long as you can maintain some sort of a job and feed, clothe, and house yourself. The rest is optional. It is indeed a wonderful feeling to be appreciated and admired. But, ironically, if you *demand* that you be competent at all times, you won't even be able to enjoy your moments of glory! You will be thinking, "This time I did well, but next time I'll screw up and they'll find out my incompetency." So, if you change your unrealistic expectations of yourself, you won't put yourself down. Your best course of action is to calmly and consistently keep trying to do your best, forgive yourself for mistakes or delays, and try to enjoy yourself in the meanwhile.

If you have irrational demands on yourself, you may well have demands on your co-workers as well:

"I *shouldn't* have to put up with this kind of treatment!"

"My efforts *must* be recognized and justly rewarded!"

"Poor me, I *should* be treated fairly!"

"You are a no-good s--t for criticizing me!"

If you view a reprimand from your boss as a tragedy and as proof that you are totally incompetent, and if you think that the boss is the devil incarnate for having done such a thing, you will react to that reprimand in extreme ways. Emotionally you will feel any combination of anger, anxiety, and depression. Behaviorally, you may further compromise your situation by throwing a temper tantrum, quitting the job, or simply not asserting yourself and explaining why you did what you did.

On the other hand, if you view the reprimand more realistically as (a) a normal part of being employed, (b) probably a criticism of a particular act or series of acts, rather than of your personhood, and (c) the boss's right to be unreasonable at times, your emotions will be appropriate. Emotionally, you will feel disappointed and frustrated about being reprimanded. Behaviorally, you will choose a sensible course of action, such as listening carefully and trying to comply with the boss's request, or eventually even quitting, if it becomes clear that the amount of frustration this particular boss elicits is more than is worth bearing.

Being Out of Work

When you are out of work, you no longer have to put up with those unreasonable bosses and co-workers. The problem is that there are bills to pay, resumes to write, interviews to hope to get and live through. Being out of work has encouraged many people to overeat, drink, or engage in whatever vice they favor. Irrational ideas abound:

"If I were a competent worker, I wouldn't be in this position. I'm clearly a loser."

"How could people be so cruel?"

"The world is obviously rotten and unfair for me to be in this situation, and it *shouldn't* be!"

"Things will *never* go well for me."

"I'll never get a job I want, and if I do I'm sure I won't keep it."

"I *can't stand* writing all these resumes, making all these phone calls. I can't bear another rejection."

"I *need* the certainty of a weekly paycheck."

"I *need* to know what will happen to me. I *can't stand* the suspense!"

Unemployment happens, even to competent people. It is unpleasant, but sometimes it is part of your life. Perhaps you were fired with good reason. If so, learn from your mistakes, try not to repeat them. Perhaps you were unfairly fired or laid off, which is unfortunate, but with perseverance you can find yourself a new position. In the meanwhile, you can enjoy some of your off time, but mostly you can benefit from making looking for a job a full-time job itself. The more time you spend on job-search related activities, the higher your chances of getting something. It is highly unlikely that you will "never get a job." It is also very likely that you will get a number of rejections en route. If you "can't stand" rejection, or the possibility that you might make a fool of yourself at an interview, you will procrastinate. You will sit at home, feel sorry for yourself, and perhaps overeat. But if you allow for some rejections and for some poor interviews, you will keep at it until a reasonably appropriate job is offered to you, and you will spend less time (and money) indulging in food.

13

To Lose or Not to Lose: Making Rational Decisions

In previous chapters, we have presented different views of fatness, and we have showed that fat is not inherently evil and undesirable. How much of it is considered desirable varies from person to person and culture to culture. Further, for some individuals within each culture, weight simply is not an important consideration, be it above or below the social ideal.

It is important that you see and fully accept that standards are subjective, and, except for ways in which your fatness may be affecting your health, it is not objectively wrong, sinful, or unacceptable. We can also note that, on the average, if your weight is above your society's ideal, it can be an obstacle in obtaining others' personal and professional level interest. Not an insurmountable obstacle, but an obstacle nevertheless. If you want to achieve intimate relationships and career success, being fashionably thin is helpful in our society. If you are not, you will have to work extra hard to achieve the same goals.

An important question to answer is, are you really overweight? A 1985 survey indicated that ninety percent of Americans think they weigh too much. On any day,

twenty-five percent of us are on diets, and another fifty
percent are in-between diets. Some of these dieters indeed weigh too much for their health. Others diet only
because our society has settled on an ideal that can only be
achieved by drastically restricting food intake and/or exercising frequently.

At some point a person is no longer at his ideal
weight, he is overweight. That point is an elusive one, and
so is the distance from that point at which one should be
concerned about this extra weight. As we have mentioned
before, everyone has their own ideal weight in terms of
health, according to their predisposition, and metabolic
rate. Because it is so hard to know what amount of fat is
healthy for each person, we tend to think in simplistic
terms: fat is bad, so the less of it we have, the better.
Fashion certainly dictates this idea. But because being
really overweight is not good or healthy, does it follow that
having *any* fat is also bad? Obviously adipose tissue is
a necessary part of the human body. Very underweight
women do not menstruate, and cannot bear children. Few
of us consider being "skin and bones" desirable.

Aside from dealing with the ideal weight in terms of
health, we come to the issue of attractiveness. At what
weight are *you* at your best? We have already determined
that thin is fashionable, and that you may look more attractive if you lose weight. But not necessarily. An example of
someone who lost weight as well as looks is Emilia. You
may be able to think of others like her. Emilia is very
attractive, and also only slightly chubby. Marital problems
gave her the incentive to control what she could, her
eating. She enrolled in a weight loss program, and lost
twenty-one pounds, a rather large amount for her five foot
four inch frame. She was proud of her accomplishment,
but in reality she became somewhat less attractive at her
new "fashionable weight." Her body lost its curves and
became more boyish, and her head now seemed a bit too

large for her frame. She received compliments on her self-control, on her ability to lose weight, but some male friends noted that she used to be sexier.

You may be different from Emilia, you may look better at a lower weight. But often the problem isn't only how much you weigh. Rather, your adipose tissue may refuse to distribute itself quite as you'd like it. It "sticks out" in places, does not conform to the smooth lines of our modern tailored clothing. Fat has a life of its own—you gain in some spots, not in others, and when you lose, you often lose it from places from which you'd better not lose. A hospital administrator one of the authors once worked with was not fat, but heavier than she would have liked to be, and she was able to rapidly lose about twenty-five pounds. Everyone complimented her greatly, because when her fat was gone, an unusually symmetrical and aesthetically pleasing, thin-waisted figure emerged.

This example is notable because of its unusualness. Very few persons who lose weight uncover such a pleasing figure as this administrator. More typically, an average-looking, chubby woman who loses some weight becomes an average looking thinner woman. One client, Sylvia, also only mildly overweight, was after many attempts finally able to control her weight, and lost twenty-two pounds. At her new weight, she often experienced hunger pangs and some weakness. At five foot eleven and 142 pounds, she was not underweight by most standards, except apparently by her own internal setpoint.

Sylvia felt she could live with the hunger pangs and weakness, and was very pleased at first with her new look. Her dimensions approached those of a fashion model—tall and slender. But slowly she noted that although the weight loss was welcome on most of her parts, she missed her large, sexy breasts, which had become much less impressive. She had also liked her face a little rounder. She did receive many compliments on her new weight (it occurs to

very few people to question whether weight loss could
ever be detrimental to one's looks), however, she did not
find that men were any more attracted to her than before.
She decided to gain some of the weight back, trying to find
a weight where the appearance of her face, breasts, and
hips were optimized. There was no real ideal weight for
her that could make all her parts ideally proportioned. Her
genes dictated that the thinner the thighs, the flatter her
chest. Like millions of others, she had to choose, or to
compromise.

Many women learn to see their bodies as objects, to
be molded according to external standards. This is in some
respects a rational response to external pressures, because
looking a certain "acceptable" way usually does help bring
desired results in personal and professional relationships.
Good appearance helps one's social standing, particularly
for women. But thinking of one's body solely in terms of
whether or not it pleases others means forgetting about the
ultimate reason for wanting to please them in the first
place—that is, personal happiness and well-being. It
means jumping from the *desire* to the *demand* to be pleasant looking. A naturally fat person who has this demand
will either severely blame herself for not meeting it, or will
starve herself to the point of feeling weak and unhealthy,
and then perhaps binge and feel even worse about herself.

Looking at it from the point of view of social acceptance alone, being at peace with yourself, and having
energy and a pleasant disposition will help you be liked
much more than simply weighing twenty pounds less.
Looking at the whole picture of what you have to offer
overall, weight is just one item. Your goal preferably
should be to establish a sense of body and self- acceptance
not based on appearances. If you cannot be of average
weight without self-starvation, think of your body for what
it can do for you: it is large, noticeable, important. Keep
it in shape. Being fat does not have to mean being out

of shape. Strength is an attractive attribute in men and women of all sizes.

Everybody and every body is different. Before mass manufacturing of clothes began, tailors did not expect one person's clothes to fit another. Various shapes and sizes were expected and accepted then to a much larger extent than they are today. Modern fashion industry has found a way to fit most people into standardized sizes. However, these standard sizes in turn have created a demand that we fit them.

In the light of our society's rigid views of what is "normal," more than thirty percent of American women wear a size sixteen or larger dress.[1] But we consider anything over size fourteen to be a "large" size, as opposed to a "normal" size. One-third of American women have been deemed abnormal through this definition! We confuse what "should" be "normal" with what is actually the norm or average—so that one-third of our female population ends up as "abnormal"! We are so indoctrinated with slender beauties in the media that we get our percentages confused. We come to think that these exceptional women are the norm, or close to it. If you are a size sixteen or eighteen, you can legitimately choose to think of yourself as "normal." Clearly, you are not unusual. Perhaps if you take this attitude, others will catch on as well.

Spot reducing does not work. You can build muscles in a certain part of your body, but the fat above it will not come off any quicker than the fat on your body overall.[2] Though diet and exercise can help improve your appearance, for most people the search for a "perfect" body is doomed from the start. Some of you may be disappointed about this state of affairs, but accept it and go on with your lives. Others, especially women, often decide that it is "awful" not to have a perfect body, that they cannot truly enjoy their lives until they do. But since the great majority of human beings have at least some minor deformities and imperfections, are they not then dooming much of the human race to misery?

It is simply a matter of re-adjusting your focus and accepting imperfections without being miserable about them. Aside from winning beauty contests, there are very few pleasurable activities in life that could not be enjoyed with an imperfect body. And even most of the beauty queens soon get "too fat"!

How Much to Work on that LFT

With the abundance and variety of food surrounding us and the largely sedentary life most of us lead, exerting some control over our food intake is highly desirable. But must we be as thin as high fashion dictates in order to enjoy life? Equally important, can we enjoy life in a state of constant starvation? This may be a case of losing sight of the forest for the trees. We set out to lose weight in order to be happier, but the constant deprivation and self-downing for not achieving our ideal weight goal often makes us miserable.

An eastern European-born author writing about eating disorders in Western culture [3] describes how she thinks of her body in terms of what her body is able to do, not how it appears: "Most of my waking life I am hardly aware of my body . . . I become aware of my body when I realize I am hungry or thirsty or have to go to the washroom . . . when my back is hurting, I may be annoyed with the body I have. I am pleasantly aware of my body when I take a long walk or swim or do some physical work or activity . . . I eat when I am hungry . . . and then forget about food. My body is not the focus of my attention, unless it prevents me from engaging in an activity I want to pursue."

The constant dieter often forgets that her body is there to help her do things and feel good, not just to convey a certain look. It is always good to have high frustration tolerance, but perhaps concentrating all or most of your energies on this one, albeit reasonable, goal of losing weight, will not leave you much energy and creativity left for more meaningful activities. Our bodies' primary function is, after all, to carry us through the day. The stronger and healthier it feels, the better it will serve us.

A certain amount of self-deprivation is an appropriate part of life. You are surrounded by tempting food choices, and eating everything that seems appealing will not only make you fat, but will also make you feel sick and weak. Being a long-term as well as a short-term hedonist maximizes your enjoyment of life by striking a balance between self-indulgence and self-deprivation. Reality says that you cannot have it all—cannot have that cake and be thin too. And perhaps you as an individual cannot be fashionably thin and have energy as well. This is not awful or terrible though. It is a situation in which you have choices. To diet or not to diet? How much to diet? You decide, and whatever you choose is a valid choice. Even if it has real disadvantages.

Self-Acceptance

As fallible human beings, we can work on being able to tolerate frustration (such as hunger) better, but we'll never be comfortable with it. As mentioned earlier, research shows that bingeing after severe restriction of food intake is the body's natural attempt to try to reinstate equilibrium. By choosing to like and accept ourselves conditionally, on the basis of being totally in control of our food intake, most of us will hate ourselves.

Choosing to target a weight below the weight your body comfortably maintains means constant work and vigilance. With controlling your weight, just as in the professional world and in personal relationships, sometimes you do better than other times. No one will deny that it is good to try to reach and maintain a target weight, to excel at work, and to maintain positive relationships in your life. It is good to work as hard as you can at these goals, and to find creative ways of achieving them. It is good because these goals have advantages, not because they will make you feel good about yourself.

Ultimately you are the one making yourself feel good about yourself. Just as you can say "I like myself because I accomplished X, Y and Z," you can decide to say "I like myself because I am me, my own most precious possession." The latter is preferable because it is unconditional, it is safe, and it can *always* be achieved. It is a starting point for working at creating a life that is pleasing to you. The more you achieve, the more pleased you can be about your *achievements*, but never about *yourself*.

Yes, you *can* stand not having it all. It would be nice to have it all, but it doesn't have to be that way. Further, you can stand yourself even if you are far from perfect (which you are, and that's OK!). Accepting yourself is a choice, just like hating yourself is a choice. Your chances of being successful at anything are much higher if you are comfortable with yourself, self-accepting. The ultimate reason for losing weight is to improve the quality of your life, to enjoy it more. But by only *conditionally* accepting yourself ("I will only be OK if I lose the damned weight") and by lambasting yourself for your imperfections, you significantly and unnecessarily lower the quality of your life.

In the previous chapters we talked about the many factors that influence how much each individual weighs, factors that influence how this weight is perceived, and what the ideal weight is for each person from a physiological point of view. For those of us with a genetically high setpoint, keeping our weight at today's societal ideal will involve a great deal of effort and self-denial. Though it is certainly do-able, you might well decide that it is not worthwhile. The health risks of yo-yoing back and forth are also to be considered as a negative aspect of deciding to aim at a weight lower than that which is comfortable for your body.

Keeping in mind the big picture, the fact that losing weight is a means towards improving the quality of your life, you can ask yourself again: "How much of the quality of my life am I giving up by constantly dieting? Perhaps I should settle for a goal weight which is a little higher than what I would ideally prefer, so that I will not have to restrict my food intake quite so drastically."

Many factors will influence each person's equation. Everyone has different contingencies, such as different people in their lives who feel differently about weight, or different jobs which may or may not require a slender figure. If your reason for wanting to lose weight is to find a mate, an option might be to spend more time and effort meeting partners who might be interested in your present weight. As mentioned earlier, you can become involved with the National Association for the Advancement of Fat Acceptance (NAAFA).

Once you give up absolutistic demands and achieve unconditional self-acceptance, you can then go on and realistically judge the pluses and minuses of maintaining different weight levels as well as making other life choices. Then decide on a liveable weight and life.

You may want to think about the fact that in today's society, too much creativity and energy go into the goal of thinness—fitting into the standard sizes, looking inoffensive and pleasing to as many people as possible. Even in times of economic recession, we are relatively very rich as a society. With this well-being seems to come the values of personal achievement and success, as shown by money, power and sex. One of women's main goals is to be physically attractive, to fit the description of the wife or girlfriend of a successful male, one who can "buy" an attractive woman. Perhaps if we were more concerned with things outside of ourselves, such as politics, work, or helping the poor in this and other countries, our specific shape would be less important. The energy that many of us now spend on perfecting our bodies could be put to much better use, not only in helping others, but in broadening our horizons and achieving the inner beauty that will attract other non-shallow persons.

The world is so far from being perfect that many religious philosophers are pondering why a kind God would have placed us in such a terrible place, or allowed things to get this bad without intervening. But what many American and other Western middle-class or upper-class persons are doing is ignoring reality, and trying to create the illusion of perfection with their lives and looks. Having that ideal thin body supposedly shows that one's life is perfect, under control. But how often is it, really?

All is certainly not well in the world, and even within each of our lives there are always problems. There is no real need to pretend otherwise. Excellence in some area(s) is often within our reach, but perfection never is. Perhaps a synonym for "human" is "imperfect." It is also human nature to strive for more: more accomplishments, more possessions. This is quite healthy, because hard work will improve our lives, and it is simply fun to learn new things and reach new levels of competence.

But being thin is not much of an achievement—it is just the absence of something we consider undesirable—fat. Few people will feel happy and fulfilled in life simply because they are not fat. On the other hand, plenty of people have managed to lead fascinating, fulfilling lives, even though they were fat or their appearance was otherwise not at the height of fashion. Creative geniuses do not strive for perfection, nor do they strive to fit a common standard. Rather, they mostly strive to develop their own inner potential, and use their unique approach to solve a previously unsolved problem or to give the world a different outlook (as in arts). You may also consider putting more energy into creative pursuits. In doing so, you may even be pleasantly surprised to find that having a creative, vitally absorbing interest will help you to more effortlessly lose some weight.

Notes for Chapter 13.

1. DuCoff & Cohen, 1980.
2. Rodin, Radke Sharpe, Rebuffe Scrive & Greenwood, 1990.
3. Szekely, 1988.

14

Cognitive Methods of Overcoming Emotional Problems

As we have emphasized in this book, fatness itself is usually not an eating disorder and does not result from or go with any serious personality disorder. But sometimes it does. People may overeat (like they drink, drug, gamble, or smoke too much) because of their anxiety, depression, self-hatred, rage, low frustration tolerance, or obsessive-compulsiveness.

Fat people, as we have also shown, may be perfectionistic about their weight, may put themselves down for weighing "too much," may have low frustration about the hassles of being chubby, and may have other emotional problems about weight and other life issues. Anorectics, bulimics, and other people with eating disorders, as we have again demonstrated, almost always are disturbed.

This book would therefore hardly be complete unless we indicated how you can use RET to overcome your emotional problems about eating or anything else. So we shall present, in this and the next two chapters, some of the most popular RET techniques, especially those that can be used for self-help purposes. We shall apply these methods particularly to eating problems but you can use them to help yourself with other thinking, feeling, and behavioral disturbances. We shall now summarize and repeat the RET techniques we have previously mentioned and shall add other popular RET methods that we have not already covered.[1]

Disputing Your Irrational Beliefs: Disputing Demandingness

We have given a good many examples of Disputing (D) your irrational Beliefs (iBs) in previous chapters, but let us briefly review this very important method again. Whenever you are disturbed—or, more accurately stated, *disturb yourself*—about anything, you largely do so by taking your rational or appropriate *preferences* and *desires* and making them into absolutistic demands: *musts, shoulds, oughts, necessities*, and other *imperatives*. Thus, you take your *preferences* for proper eating and weight and irrationally insist:

"I *must* weigh 30 pounds less than I do now!"

"I *absolutely should* not gain any more weight!"

"I always *have to* keep strictly on my diet!"

"I've *got to* be perfectly thin at all times!"

"If I eat any extra food, I completely *need* to purge myself immediately so that I will gain no weight."

"It is *imperative* that people approve of me."

To Dispute these unrealistic and illogical demands, you actively *look for* and *find* them, when you are disturbed and you use the scientific method to question and challenge them, until you change them back into preferences:[1,2]

Disputing: "Why *must* I weigh thirty pounds less than I now do?"

Rational Answer: "There is *no* reason why I must, though it would be preferable if I did. I would really *like to* lose it but I don't *have to* do so."

Disputing: "Where is the evidence that I *absolutely should not* gain any more weight?"

Rational Answer: "There isn't any. There is evidence that it might be desirable if I gained no more weight, but it doesn't follow that therefore I *absolutely should* not."

Disputing: "In what way do I always *have to* keep strictly on my diet?"

Rational Answer: "In no way! I'd *like to* but of course I never *have to*."

Disputing: "Is there really any reason why I've *got to* be perfectly thin at all times?"

Rational Answer: "Of course not! I'll never be perfectly anything, including perfectly thin. Even if I could be, there's no reason why I've *got* to be."

Disputing: "Prove that if I eat any extra food, I completely *need* to purge myself immediately so that I will gain no weight."

Rational Answer: "Nonsense! No matter how much extra food I eat, and no matter how much I *want* to lose weight immediately, I don't *need* to purge myself. I can slowly diet, if I decide to do so, to stop the effects of my bingeing. Or I can forget about this meal and stay away from extra food in the future."

Disputing: "Where is it written that it is *imperative* that people approve of me?"

Rational Answer: "Only in my nutty head. It would be lovely if significant people approved of me. But that never makes it *imperative* or necessary!"

Margaret strongly believed that she *must not*, in spite of her six feet two inches height, weigh more than 120 pounds, that she *absolutely should* be depressed about her

usual weight of 145 pounds, and that she *had to* purge
every time she even moderately "overate." When she gave
up these *demands* she still weighed 145 pounds (and sometimes more) but was no longer depressed or purging.

Disputing Awfulizing

As we have also noted in this book, once you demand
that something *must* or *must not* be a certain way, and in
reality it isn't the way it *absolutely should* be, you tend to
awfulize about it:

> "Because I weigh thirty pounds more than I *must*
> weigh, it's *awful!*"

> "I *absolutely should not* gain any more weight and I
> actually *have* gained five more pounds, and that is
> *terrible!*"

> "As I always *have to* strictly stay on my diet and I have
> *not* done so, it's *horrible.*"

> "I've *got to* be perfectly thin at all times and I've just
> gained three pounds. How awful!"

> "It's *terrible and horrible* when I eat extra food and I
> fail to purge immediately as I *must* do to avoid gaining
> any weight!"

> "It's *imperative* that people approve of me, so it's
> *horrible* when they don't!"

Awfulizing is wrong and self-defeating because if
something were really *awful* or *terrible* it would be (1)
totally, one hundred percent bad; (2) more than bad; and
(3) badder than it *should be*—that is, it should be less bad
than it actually is and because it isn't less bad than it must
be, it's *awful!* You can actively find and Dispute your
awfulizing as follows:

Disputing: "Why is it *awful* or *terrible* to gain any weight, to even slightly go off my diet, to fail to be perfectly thin, to fail to purge when I eat extra food, or to have people disapprove of me?"

Rational Answer: "It never is *awful* or *terrible*, however bad and uncomfortable I may find these things. At worst, it's highly inconvenient but hardly the end of the world or the end of my life in this world!"

Josephina felt it was *awful and terrible* when her parents kept insisting—rightly!—that she looked like a skeleton and might well kill herself when she starved herself down to seventy-eight pounds. When she was shown, in RET sessions, that nothing is really awful, but at worst only inconvenient, she stopped hating her parents and managed to put forty more pounds on her five feet four frame. She didn't like her new "fatness" but didn't view it as *awful*.

Disputing I-can't-stand-it-itis

I-can't-stand-it-itis, usually leading to low frustration tolerance or discomfort disturbance, is common among overweight people and those with eating disorders. It stems from irrational Beliefs (iBs) like these:

"Because I *must* weigh thirty pounds less and I don't, *I can't stand it!*"

"I *absolutely should* never gain more weight, and I actually have gained five more pounds, and *I can't bear it!*"

"As I always *have to* strictly stay on my diet and I have not done so, *I can't tolerate* going off it!"

"When I eat extra food, as I *must* not, *I can't stand* not purging, so I *have* to purge!"

"I *can't bear* people disapproving of me because it is *imperative* that they like me!"

I-can't-stand-it-itis is a false position, because if you really *couldn't stand* something you would die of its existence, or it would be impossible for you to live and be happy *at all.* You can Dispute all your I-can't-stand-its as follows:

Disputing: "Why can't I stand weighing thirty pounds more than I'd like to weigh?"
Rational Answer: "I'll never like weighing so much but I *can* stand it and still lead a happy life."

Disputing: "Why *must* I never gain more weight, and where is the evidence that I *can't bear it* if I do?"
Rational Answer: "There is no reason, of course, why I must never gain more weight and no evidence that I *can't stand it* if I do. I *can* stand what I don't like!"

Disputing: "Prove that I *can't* tolerate going off my diet."
Rational Answer: "Of course I can tolerate it, even though I'll get bad results by going off it. I won't die of these results and can still be happy in spite of them."

Disputing: "In what way do I *have to* be perfectly thin at all times and *can't stand* gaining three pounds?"
Rational Answer: "In *no* way! I *can* stand gaining weight. I still dislike it, but I can live with it!"

Disputing: "When I eat too much, why can't I *stand* not purging and *stand* regular dieting instead?"
Rational Answer: "I damned well *can* stand regular dieting instead of purging. And I'd better!"

Disputing: "In what manner can't I *bear* the discomfort and pain of significant people not liking me?"

Rational Answer: "I can not only *bear* it, but I can also determine why they don't like me—or like what I do—and probably get more of them to like me. If not, I can still lead a happy life, though not as happy as if I have more good friends."

Mabelline and Robert, a husband and wife, just *couldn't stand* food that was not organically grown and were having a hard time, in their small town, getting such food. When they decided, mainly by reading and listening to RET materials, that they *could* stand what they didn't like, they made some food compromises, their life became much easier, and they stopped being so severely anxious.

Disputing Self-Downing

Self-downing or *self*-hatred, over and above criticizing some of your *characteristics*, is perhaps the worst form of emotional disturbance. It often helps drive people to over-eating, and then zaps them *for* their consequent "fatness." You, like millions of people, can easily lambaste yourself for being "overweight," for gaining more weight (even when you are slender), for going off your diet, for not being *perfectly* thin, for bingeing and *not* resorting to purging, for not being loved by significant people, and for *any other* failure you think you have. According to RET, all *self*-blaming (instead of merely criticizing some of your behaviors) is incorrect and anxiety-producing, and is to be actively and forcefully Disputed. For example:

Disputing: "Where is the proof that *I*, as a *person*, am rotten or worthless when I am too heavy, when I gain more weight, when I go off my diet, when I fail to make myself *perfectly* thin, when I binge and fail to purge myself, when I am disapproved of by significant people, or when I do *anything* badly or foolishly?"

Rational Answer: "Nowhere! The "proof" of *me* being rotten or worthless is nonexistent. I *do* many stupid, self-defeating *acts* and, as a fallible human, will always do some more. But I am only a *person who* does these things, never a *bad person*! I can usually change my poor eating and other habits. But if I never do, I can still always accept *myself*, my *personhood*, and I still deserve to make myself as happy as I can."

Maryanne hated herself for hating herself. She originally lambasted herself for her being, according to her ideal goals, thirty-five pounds overweight. But then, learning some RET, she realized that self-hatred was stupid, and probably helped her *gain* weight, so she loathed herself for her self-loathing. She was a difficult customer (DC) in therapy, because she seemed to *want* to hate herself for *something*, and what was better than severely castigating herself for downing herself? Nothing! She finally was able to convince herself, "*All* self-downing is indeed stupid. So I'd better stop it! But I never will if I keep downing myself! So I'm determined to give that up *first*!" She worked hard with her RET, and actually did accept herself—but not what she *did*—when she put herself down. Once she accomplished that, as she put it, "the rest is easy. I now have no trouble at all accepting myself, even liking myself, in spite of my overeating."

Disputing Allness and Neverness and Black and White Thinking

People with eating problems, and just about all humans, often think in terms of allness and neverness and wrongly convince themselves that they have to *always* act poorly, can *never* change, and are one hundred percent "good" or "bad" in their deeds and traits. And what dismal emotional and behavioral problems, about eating and everything else, they then create! When you do this kind of all or nothing thinking about dieting and other problems, you can Dispute it as follows:

Disputing: "Why will I *never* be able to lose weight, to eat proper foods, to stop bingeing, or to quit purging when I binge?"

Rational Answer: "I'd better never say never to having these difficulties. I may always have trouble losing weight, eating properly, stopping bingeing, and quitting purging when I binge. But that doesn't mean that I *never* can do so. Of course, I may never achieve an *ideal* weight or figure. Too bad! I can accept that and still lead a happy life."

Disputing: "Do I really have to *always* be thin, *always* keep perfectly to my diet, *always* purge when I binge, *always* be loved by significant people?"

Rational Answer: "Of course not! The only thing I'll probably always be is a highly *fallible* human. Therefore, I may well *often* eat badly and turn some people off. But if I keep trying, I can also *often* eat well and win the approval of significant others. But not *always!*"

Disputing: "Why are my eating habits *totally* bad? Why must I never ingest *any* undesirable food? Why must I *completely* be approved by my friends and family members?"

Rational Answer: "For no reason! I can allow myself *some* poor eating habits and *some* undesirable food. I'd *like* to be completely approved by my friends and family members, but that is highly improbable. I can be happy with *some* of their approval and even refuse to make myself miserable when they disapprove of me."

William procrastinated on almost everything—especially on mapping out a healthy diet and sticking to it. "I *never* do anything on time!" he kept saying to his RET group. "I *always* screw things up. So I'm a *real, total* screw-up!" But the group pointed out to him that he did a good many things quite well, including helping other group members with their RET. William finally agreed with them and started saying, "Yes, I'd better admit that I *often* procrastinate, *frequently* screw up, and *rarely* stick to my diet. But not *always*. Even I am not *that much* of a screw-up. Largely, but not *totally*!" His self-downing then stopped. He hardly became a perfect dieter but did much better at eating healthy foods.

Coping Self-Statements

As we have previously noted, when you give yourself rational answers to your Disputing questions, you can write some of these on a three by five card, carry them with you, and go over and *think* about (not parrot) them several times a day, until you start to automatically believe them and act on them.[2,4] For example, you can use coping self-statements like these:

"I *can*, probably, lose some more weight as long as I am realistic about my body's tendency to be chubby. But I never *have to* lose it and can accept myself at *any* weight!"

"Weighing more than I would like to weigh is unfortunate and has real disadvantages. But it's not *awful or horrible*, only inconvenient!"

"I *can stand* going off my diet but I'll never *prefer* it. So back to the drawing board, to see how well I can do to stay on it."

"My being approved by significant others is really important to me. But I can always decide to do a much more important thing: unconditionally *accept myself*, just because I *choose* to do so, *whether or not* I act well and *whether or not* other people approve of me!"

Referenting

When you are emotionally disturbed you tend to referent—or one-sidedly refer in your mind to—mainly the *advantages* of your self-defeating behavior (such as the advantages of overeating, bingeing, starving yourself, smoking, and overdrinking). And you referent or focus on mainly the *disadvantages* of disciplining yourself and forcing yourself to engage in self-helping behavior (such as dieting, non-bingeing, and abstinence from smoking and problem drinking).

Following some of the principles of general semantics, RET teaches people to referent the *disadvantages* of their self-defeating behavior and also to referent the *advantages* of their self-helping actions.[3,5] To do this, you take an undesired behavior, such as bingeing, and for two or three weeks you make a long list of its *disadvantages*—for example, gaining weight, resorting to harmful purging, sabotaging your health, turning off other people, etc. Carry this list with you and go over it and *think about it* several times every day, until you automatically keep it in mind and start acting on it.

You can also make a list of the *advantages* of desirable behavior, such as steady dieting—for example, health benefits, good discipline, avoidance of bingeing and purging, getting more approval from friends and supervisors, etc. Again, forcefully go over this list several times a day until you sink it into your head and heart and actually begin to diet steadily.

Similarly, you can referent the many benefits of unconditionally accepting yourself and the many *liabilities* of putting yourself down, and persistently think about them until you achieve much more self-acceptance.

Thelma could see almost no advantages, and many disadvantages, in keeping her five feet four frame below 180 pounds. Her physician insisted that she do so or she would have to resort to taking insulin for her Type 2 (non-insulin-dependent) Diabetes. But she said she'd rather continue her high-fat diet and take the insulin.

Her RET group, which she was attending mainly because of her loneliness, urged her to do more referenting, and she finally reluctantly did it. To her surprise, she came up with a list of seventeen advantages of dieting, including better health, improved appearance, more dating possibilities, fewer fights with her mother and brother, better job possibilities, and more energy. After going over this list five times a day for two weeks, she began to follow her doctor's dieting directions.

Teaching Others RET

Just as AA (and other twelve-step programs) and Rational Recovery programs encourage their members to spread the word and teach non-members their principles, so does RET encourage you to learn the techniques outlined in this book and to teach them to your (unsuspecting or suspecting!) friends and relatives. The more you teach others the ABC's of RET and how to Dispute (D) their irrational Beliefs (iBs), the more you may help them—and the more you will most likely help yourself to get these principles and practices into your own head and to use them steadily yourself.[6]

Cyril said that he was "too lazy" to do much RET Disputing about his *need* to eat all night while watching television after having eaten carefully all day. He accepted the homework assignment, however, of finding several people with similar "needs" and with other so called "necessities" and talking them out of their necessitizing. Following this assignment, he began to strongly talk several of his friends out of their dire "needs" for food, for love, for success, and for other things. He soon changed his "necessity" for food (and for love) into a strong preference and kept his after-dinner eating to a minimum.

Modeling and Mentoring

As Albert Bandura and other psychologists have pointed out, children and adults learn a good deal from modeling. So if you want to help yourself think rationally, feel appropriately, and behave effectively, try to find some friends or relatives who do well in these ways and work at modeling yourself after them.[6,7] If you have trouble finding a good model, consider joining a suitable therapist, therapy group, or self-help group where you can find good models.

Good mentors are also usually hard to locate, but you may be able to find a few wise and experienced individuals who are willing to teach you some of their philosophies, skills, and methods of self-discipline. Don't take any of these mentors too seriously or worship them, but selectively use what help you can from their teachings.

Saul was doing poorly with his dieting, and was eating sugary foods that seemed to affect him badly and help make him unduly enraged at strangers whom he thought were acting badly. But he was doing so well with his Alcoholics Anonymous sponsor who helped him keep sober that he decided to find a mentor outside of AA who would supervise his eating. One of his co-workers took on the job and with this person's help and supervision, Saul was able to stay away from all sweets.

Use of Accurate Language

Alfred Korzybski and some of his main students, such as Wendell Johnson, S.I. Hayakawa, and D. David Bourland, have pioneered in demonstrating that our crooked thinking gets into and produces overgeneralized language, and that this language, in turn, leads to more distorted thinking, inappropriate feeling, and ineffective behavior.[5,8] To change this, watch your language! Check what you say to yourself and others, see how misleading some of your language is, and keep changing it until you rarely fall prey to it. Here are some examples of what to look for and change:

Overgeneralized statement: "I *am* a poor dieter."
Less disturbing alternative: "I often diet poorly but at times I eat well and *can* diet better now and in the future.

Inaccurate statement: "People make me angry and drive me to overeating."
Less disturbing alternative: "People sometimes act poorly but I choose to tell myself that they *must not* act that way. I therefore *make myself* angry at them. Then I *choose* to drive myself to overeating."

Overgeneralized statement: "Eating poorly and stupidly makes me a rotten, stupid person!"
Less disturbing alternative: "Eating poorly and stupidly makes me a *person who* is *now* behaving poorly and who can change and eat better in the future.

Overgeneralized statement: "Because I've fallen back from my diet many times, *it's hopeless*, and I'll *never* be able to keep eating properly."
Less disturbing alternative: "Because I've fallen back from my diet many times, *I find it difficult* to keep eating properly. But that doesn't mean it's hopeless or impossible. I'll keep trying!"

Reading and Listening to RET Materials

In using RET, the authors of this book have found that our clients who read the RET literature, listen to RET audio and video cassettes, and go to lectures and workshops at the Institute for Rational-Emotive Therapy in New York and other parts of the world, usually learn and use RET better than those who do not do this kind of reading and listening. Several studies of RET and other self-help materials, moreover, have shown that with and without psychotherapy people can significantly change themselves when they use these materials.[9]

We suggest, therefore, that you make good use of some of the RET reading and listening materials listed at the back of this book, most of which can be obtained from the Institute for Rational-Emotive Therapy, 45 East 65th Street, New York, NY 10021-6593. If you have specific eating and other addiction problems, we recommend these books and pamphlets: A. Ellis, & E. Velten, *When AA Doesn't Work For You: Rational Steps to Quitting Alcohol*; J. Trimpey, *Rational Recovery From Alcoholism: The Small Book*; L. Trimpey, & J. Trimpey, *Rational Recovery From Fatness*; A. Ellis, J. McInerney, R. DiGiuseppe, & R. Yeager, *Rational-Emotive Therapy With Alcoholics and Substance Abusers*.[10] Also, these cassettes: A. Ellis, *Conquering Low Frustration Tolerance, I'd Like To Stop, But . . . Overcoming Addictions*.[11]

If you want to use RET with your general emotional problems, we recommend these books and pamphlets: A. Ellis, *Reason and Emotion in Psychotherapy; How to Live With a "Neurotic"*; A. Ellis & I. Becker, *A Guide to Personal Happiness*; A. Ellis, *Anger: How To Live With and Without It*; P. Jakubowski & A. Lange, *The Assertive Option*; D. Burns, *Feeling Good*; P.A. Hauck, *Overcoming Depression*; H. Young, *Rational Counseling Primer*; A. Ellis, *How To Stubbornly Refuse to Make Yourself Miserable About Anything—Yes, Anything!*; W. Dryden, *Dealing With Your Anger Problems*; A. Ellis & R.A. Harper, *A New Guide to Rational Living*; W. Dryden & J. Gordon, *Think Your Way to Happiness*.[12] Also, these cassettes: A. Ellis, *A Garland of Rational Songs, Albert Ellis Live at the Learning Annex, Rational Living in an Irrational World, Unconditionally Accepting Yourself and Others, RET and Assertiveness Training, Twenty-Two Ways to Brighten Your Love Life*; R. DiGiuseppe, *What Do I Do With My Anger: Hold It In Or Let It Out*, W. Knaus, *Overcoming*

Procrastination; A. Ellis & R.A. Harper, *A Guide to Rational Living.* [13]

John, who was turned off sexually by his wife, Joan, because she was usually about fifty pounds more than he would have liked her to be, tried to get her into individual or group therapy, into a Rational Recovery group, or into Weight Watchers or some other reducing program. No chance! Joan had a million excuses—especially that of being too busy caring for their three young children. Seeing that none of his suggestions were working, and talking about his problem with Joan at the regular Friday Night Workshop, Problems of Everyday Living at the New York Institute for Rational-Emotive Therapy, John urged Joan to do some RET reading and cassette listening. She at first resisted this, too. But he induced her to read and listen to the materials a half-hour a day with him. This collaborative reading and listening soon caught on; and Joan then started finding time to do some of it herself. She found the RET tapes, *Conquering Low Frustration Tolerance* and *I'd Like to Stop, But . . . : Overcoming Addictions* particularly helpful. Eventually she lost forty pounds and kept it off, thus extremely pleasing John and encouraging their having a much better sex life.

Reframing

When disturbed people, including those with eating problems, look at life they tend to focus on its unfortunate Activating Events or Adversities (A's) and then blow them up, catastrophize and awfulize about them. Obviously, however, Adversities are not totally bad, but also had some advantages. If, for example, a new acquaintance rejects you it is *good* to get rid of that person who doesn't like you *fast*. So don't just focus on the "horrors" of such a loss!

In using the technique of reframing, you look for a focus on the good or advantageous aspects of your bad

Activating Events (A's) or even of your unfavorable Consequences (Cs). Thus, you recognize that overeating provides you with fine-tasting food, provides you with something to do, lets you be a gourmet cook, gives you the
challenge of eating differently, gives you the opportunity
not to put yourself down for your undisciplined behavior,
etc.

You can even find advantages in the disadvantages of
being overweight. For example, your fatness may turn off
people who would mainly like you for your looks and not
for your other traits; it can give you a feeling of solidity and
comfort; it can give you practice in unconditional self-
acceptance; it can take away the strain of your constantly
fighting against your set-point and of seriously depriving
yourself for the rest of your life; and it can be quite
attractive to some people.[14]

When you do this kind of reframing, watch your
pollyannaism and your rationalizing! If you are seriously
anorectic and in danger of starving yourself to death, you
can still unconditionally accept yourself (but not your *behavior*). However, you'd better not tell yourself that it is
good to weigh seventy pounds because some people like to
go to bed with a skeleton. Or if you are a serious binger,
you'd better not convince yourself that it is *good* to purge
because then you can get away with purging and still not
get cancer of the throat! So reframe sensibly, not foolishly!

Positive Imaging or Visualization

Emile Coué, the originator of positive thinking, also
invented the technique of positive imaging, which you
may sometimes find useful.[15] When you are discouraged
about your overeating, you can visualize yourself refusing
to eat fattening foods; you can picture yourself eating
properly and becoming thinner; you can see yourself
steadily exercising and enjoying it; you can imagine your

friends and relatives showing real pleasure at your dieting and losing weight; you can visualize potential living and sex partners favoring you because of your discipline and better looks; you can picture job interviewers taking you more seriously as you make yourself thinner, etc.

Once again, don't be unrealistic or perfectionistic in your visualizations. If as an adult you have always weighed over 160 pounds, don't visualize yourself as thin as a rail at 120 pounds! The more unrealistic your positive visualizations and your positive thoughts are, the more you will make yourself disillusioned and pessimistic. That's why Emile Coué went out of business!

Tom, who was trying to diet, had a very hard time not having a weekly dinner with his best friend, Bruce, who always insisted on their going to fine restaurants. To help himself become more assertive with Bruce, he visualized himself firmly insisting that they meet at a bar before dinner, imagined Bruce resisting and trying to induce him to go to dinner, and saw himself as assertively continuing to refuse. After much practice in this kind of visualization, Tom was able to hold his ground on several occasions, and soon Bruce agreed that they would routinely only meet for a drink and skip having dinner together.

Cognitive Homework

RET practically always gives its clients cognitive or thinking homework. Thus, the authors of this book commonly tell our clients, "Whenever you feel quite upset—such as very anxious, depressed, self-hating, or enraged—assume that you are telling yourself or thinking some absolutist shoulds, oughts, musts, demands, or commands. Look for and find these rigid demands, actively Dispute (D) and challenging them, and replace them with an Effective New Philosophy (E), which only consists of flexible (though still strong) desires and preferences.

To help you find your irrational Beliefs (iBs) and to effectively Dispute them (D), RET has designed a homework sheet that is used by clients of the Institute for Rational-Emotive Therapy in New York and that you can obtain and use to practice your own Disputing. Here is a sample RET Self-Help Report that you can use for your regular cognitive homework (pages 262–265).[16]

Cognitive Distraction

When people upset themselves about almost anything—such as fatness, thinness, or anything else—they are usually focusing on the "horror" of having or not having this thing, and thereby making themselves panicked, depressed, or enraged. As we show in this book and in other RET writings, they can almost always find their irrational Beliefs (iBs) that lead to these disturbed feelings, change them, and thereby produce appropriate instead of inappropriate feelings. But they can also temporarily distract themselves in a number of ways by strongly focusing on other things, events, conditions, or thoughts. In other words, they can use many kinds of cognitive distraction, including physical activities (such as relaxation) that include cognitive distraction.[17]

Thus, you can use Yoga, meditation, Jacobson's progressive relaxation technique, TV, other entertainment, sex, etc. to focus on *non*-panic-producing and non-depression-encouraging things and thoughts. Almost any method of cognitive distraction will work—temporarily—if you strongly and persistently use it.

Temporarily? Yes. Because if you feel horrified, for example, about your being twenty pounds overweight or underweight, you can focus on a mantra, on Yoga exercises, or on any number of relaxation methods and you will temporarily be almost incapable of worrying about, or putting you or others down about, anything.

RET SELF-HELP FORM

Institute for Rational-Emotive Therapy
45 East 65th Street, New York, NY 10021
(212) 535-0822

(A) ACTIVATING EVENTS, thoughts, or feelings that happened just before I felt emotionally disturbed or acted self-defeatingly:

(C) CONSEQUENCE OR CONDITION—disturbed feeling or self-defeating behavior—that I produced and would like to change:

(B) BELIEFS—Irrational BELIEFS (IBs) leading to my CONSEQUENCE (emotional disturbance or self-defeating behavior). Circle all that apply to these ACTIVATING EVENTS (A).	(D) DISPUTES for each circled Irrational BELIEF (iB). Examples: *"Why MUST I do very well?"* *"Where is it written* that I am a BAD PERSON?" *"Where is the evidence* that I MUST be approved or accepted?"	(E) EFFECTIVE RATIONAL BELIEFS (RBs) to replace my Irrational BELIEFS (iBs). Examples: "I'd PREFER to do very well *but I don't* HAVE TO." "I am a PERSON WHO acted badly, *not* a BAD PERSON," *"There is no evidence* that I HAVE TO to approved, though I would LIKE to be."
1. I MUST do well or very well!		
2. I am a BAD OR WORTHLESS PERSON when I act weakly or stupidly.		
3. I MUST be approved or accepted by people I find important!		
4. I NEED to be loved by someone who matters to me a lot!		
5. I am a BAD, UNLOVABLE PERSON if I get rejected.		
6. People MUST treat me fairly and give me what I NEED!		

(OVER)

262

7. People MUST live up to my expectations or it is TERRIBLE!		
8. People who act immorally are undeserving, ROTTEN PEOPLE!		
9. I CAN'T STAND really bad things or very difficult people!		
10. My life MUST have few major hassles or troubles.		
11. It's AWFUL or HORRIBLE when major things don't go my way!		
12. I CAN'T STAND IT when life is really unfair!		
13. I NEED a good deal of immediate gratification and HAVE to feel miserable when I don't get it!		
Additional Irrational Beliefs:		

(F) FEELINGS and BEHAVIORS I experience after arriving at my EFFECTIVE RATIONAL BELIEFS: _____

_____

I WILL WORK HARD TO REPEAT MY EFFECTIVE RATIONAL BELIEFS FORCEFULLY TO MYSELF ON MANY OCCASIONS SO THAT I CAN MAKE MYSELF LESS DISTURBED NOW AND ACT LESS SELF-DEFEATINGLY IN THE FUTURE.

RET SELF-HELP FORM
Institute for Rational-Emotive Therapy
45 East 65th Street, New York, NY 10021
(212) 535-0822

(A) **ACTIVATING EVENTS**, thoughts, or feelings that happened just before I felt emotionally disturbed or acted self-defeatingly:

I went off my diet and binged for two days.

(C) **CONSEQUENCE OR CONDITION** - disturbed feeling or self-defeating behavior - that I produced and would like to change:

I felt very depressed and didn't go back on my diet for a week.

(B) BELIEFS-Irrational BELIEFS (iBs) leading to my CONSEQUENCE (emotional disturbance or self-defeating behavior.) Circle all that apply to these ACTIVATING EVENTS (A)	(D) DISPUTES for each circled Irrational BELIEF (iB). Examples: "Why MUST I do very well?" "Where is it written that I am a BAD PERSON?" "Where is the evidence that I MUST be approved or accepted?"	(E) EFFECTIVE RATIONAL BELIEFS (RBs) to replace by Irrational BELIEFS (iBs). Examples: "I'd PREFER to do very well but I don't HAVE TO." "I am a PERSON WHO acted badly, not a BAD PERSON." "There is no evidence that I HAVE TO be approved, though I would LIKE to be."
1. I MUST do well or very well!	*Why must I always stick to my diet and never binge?*	*It would be great, but I don't have to always diet.*
2. I am a BAD OR WORTHLESS PERSON wehn I act weakly or stupidly.	*Does my weekly bingeing make me a weak, worthless person?*	*No, it only makes me a person who sometimes acts weakly. And who can stop doing so!*
3. I MUST be approved or accepted by people who I find important!	*Do I really have to be approved by important people for steady dieting?*	*No. I definitely want their approval, but I don't need it.*
4. I NEED to be loved by someone who matters to me a lot.		
5. I am a BAD, UNLOVABLE PERSON if I get rejected.	*If people reject me for bingeing, does that really make me a bad, unlovable person?*	*Of course not! It only makes me a person who is not loved right now.*
6. People MUST treat me fairly and give me what I NEED!		

264

7. People MUST live up to my expectations or it is TERRIBLE!

8. People who act immorally are undeserving, ROTTEN PEOPLE!

9. I CAN'T STAND really bad things or very difficult people!

How can I stand my bingeing and my depression?

By strongly believing that I _can_ stand what I don't like and can still be fairly happy.

10. My life MUST have few major hassles or troubles.

Why must I not have major hassles like steadily sticking to my diet?

No reason! It's really a hassle but bingeing only makes it worse. A hassle is not a horror!

11. It's AWFUL or HORRIBLE when major things don't go my way!

Awful? Horrible? Or just highly inconvenient?

Just highly inconvenient. Only my whining about discomforts will make them "awful."

12. I CAN'T STAND IT when life is really unfair!

Life really is unfair when I have to diet more rigorously than others do. But why can't I stand it?

I dammed well can stand it! No matter how unfair it is, I'd better put up with it.

13. I NEED a good deal of immediate gratification and HAVE to feel miserable when I don't get it!

Do I really _need_ immediate gratification?

Must I have a binge when I feel like it?

No! I'd like to gratify myself by overeating and not gaining weight. But I can't. Tough!

14. I'm no good for depressing myself.

How do I become a no-goodnik for depressing myself?

I don't. My _depression_ is bad but _I_ am not bad for foolishly bringing it on.

(F) **FEELINGS** and **BEHAVIORS** I experience after arriving at my **EFFECTIVE RATIONAL BELIEFS**: _Regret; remorse;_

disappointment; return to dieting.

I WILL WORK HARD TO REPEAT MY EFFECTIVE RATIONAL BELIEFS FORCEFULLY TO MYSELF ON MANY OCCASIONS SO THAT I CAN MAKE MYSELF LESS DISTURBED NOW AND ACT LESS SELF-DEFEATINGLY IN THE FUTURE.

Joyce Sichel, Ph.D. and Albert Ellis, Ph.D.
Copyright @ 1984 by the Institute for Rational-Emotive Therapy.

100 forms $10
1000 forms $80

265

However! Relaxation and other techniques of cognitive distraction nicely *cover up* but rarely *remove* your basic underlying irrational Beliefs (iBs) with which you keep upsetting yourself. So the *horror* of your being overweight, underweight, or anything else will soon—often very soon!—return and upset you again once you stop your relaxing and other distraction methods. So we advise our clients and readers: Whenever you feel quite upset, by all means use cognitive distraction methods; but don't stop there! After you calm yourself down, *go on* to other techniques we are describing, to non-palliatively, and sometimes permanently, uproot and change your self-defeating thoughts, feelings, and actions.

Belle became panicked whenever she thought about going to dinner with anyone and revealing that she couldn't stop bingeing on desserts and would very likely order three or four very sugary ones. So she refused all dinner invitations, especially with possible regular boyfriends. She was taught by one of the authors to use Jacobson's progressive relaxation technique, to put off potential dinner invitations, to relax, to get rid of her panic (and her panic about feeling panicked), and then to arrange for the dinner date. Until the date arrived, she then actively Disputed the irrational Beliefs (iBs) that if she revealed her bingeing to her date it would be awful and that every possible boyfriend would reject her. Doing this Disputing, she was able to have dinner dates, only occasionally eat three or four desserts, and prove to herself that she could abstain, and that when she didn't, most men thought her eating habits were cute or didn't really care that much.

Rational-Emotive Philosophy

RET assumes that there are many reasons why people are disturbed and self-defeating. But one of the most important—and changeable!—reasons is that they strongly hold unrealistic, illogical, and inflexible philosophies of life, which they tend to bring to almost everything they think, feel, and do. Therefore, if they can acquire, and really follow, a few basic self-hating philosophies, they will rarely seriously or enduringly upset themselves.[18]

Some of the basic, profound philosophies you can strive to achieve and follow—especially if you have an eating disorder or you upset yourself about your being "overweight" or "underweight"—include these:

The Philosophy of Tolerance. You don't by any means have to like or approve your or other people's behavior or what you and they think, feel, and how they and you act. But you can often give people the benefit of the doubt, assume that what they do may be legitimate or good for them (even when it isn't for *you*); and even when their behavior is generally bad and obnoxious, you can still accept or tolerate *them* while often pointing out their poor behavior. To quote the Christian philosophy, you accept the sinner but not the sin; and also try to help people behave better and sin less. Thus, you tolerate your bigoted critics, who may condemn you just because you're fat (or too thin) and you accept them *with* their bigotry, and perhaps try to induce them to be less bigoted.

The Philosophy of Acceptance. As Reinhold Niebuhr pointed out early in the 20th century, you try to have courage to change the unfortunate things you can change, the serenity to accept (but not like!) the things you can't change, and the wisdom to know the difference. Thus, if you want to lower your weight, you can do your best to eat less fattening food, to have the serenity to accept the fact that your particular set-point may limit your reaching and maintaining the ideal weight that you want, and to have the wisdom to know the difference between your *desire* and your *ability* to reach your ideal!

The Philosophy of Human Fallibility. One of the invariant facts about humans—at least so far!—is that we are all fallible; none of us is perfect or superhuman.[19] By all

means acknowledge and accept this reality! You most unlikely will be the first human who always eats perfectly,
never is a pound more or less than you would like to be,
never does foolish acts, always succeeds at important tasks,
and constantly is approved by others. Accept this "grim"
reality. Try, often, to do *your* best, or even *the* best. But
don't insist on this and never down yourself for your
inadequacies and imperfections.

The Philosophy of Interdependency. As humans,
practically all of us choose to live in a social group or
community, and we gain many advantages—and hassles!—
in doing so. So by all means try to relate to others and get
some support from them. Some! But realize that largely
you can—and had better—take care of yourself. By all
means love and help others, but don't *demand* return
support and approval. And don't expect any magical help
from higher, medium, or lower powers. If gods exist, they
most likely help those who help themselves!

You, then, will determine your weight goals, and *you*
will or will not carry them out. The hand that over- or
under-feeds you is yours! Other people and support groups
may help; and you may definitely help others with eating
and non-eating problems. So try for *mutual* support. But,
once again, don't *demand*.

Almost all humans are social animals and would hardly survive if they were not. Your very "personality," as
Edward Sampson and others have shown, is largely a social
product. Your emotional stability, as Alfred Adler pointed
out, significantly includes your *social* interest.[20] So it is not
a case of choosing *either* individual *or* social interest—but
of choosing *both*. Your goals of thinness or plumpness are
largely adapted from your culture. Your achieving these
goals largely includes *your* personal efforts—but also includes some social support. To strive for extreme independence or dependency has its real hazards. How about
some balance of interdependency and thoughtful sociality?

Sidney was so afraid of forming a lasting relationship

and losing his prized independence that he dated desirable women only once every three or four weeks, to make sure that they wouldn't get attached to him and ask him to be really involved with them. Naturally, none of his relationships lasted very long, or else turned into non-sexual friendships. In the course of twenty RET sessions, Sidney was able to see that independence was okay but had limited rewards. He took the risk of dating Joann, a new woman in his life, once or twice a week, went out of his way to ask her to help him with his social relations (which he had never done before), threw himself into helping her with her publicity business, and tried to get engaged to her. When she became seriously ill and withdrew from all social and business activities, he mourned her loss but did not make himself depressed. And instead of greatly over-eating, as he would have formerly done, he sought another independent involvement, and a year later was engaged to be married to an old friend of his with whom he had previously been unable to relate intimately. "The more I do for her," he commented, "the more I do for myself and really feel that I want to join with her. And not overeat!"

Review the Harm of Self-Rating. As we have kept showing in this book, rating your thoughts, feelings, and deeds is fine, is life-preserving, and can be very helpful; but rating your self, your being, your essence, or your personhood is not! The latter can be, and usually is, quite harmful.[21]

So review and think about the harm of self-rating. You can remind yourself, for instance:

Self-rating tends to make you anxious and panicked before an important project—unless you can guarantee you are practically perfect and will do well at all times.

It tends to help you depress yourself after you have done badly at anything.

It often deflects you from your goals and

desires—because it makes you only *want* to do what you are sure you will do *well*.

It makes you less efficient at various tasks, because you focus on "*How* am I doing? I *must* do it well enough to make me a worthy person!" instead of "*What* am I doing? Let me see if I can do it better."

Self-rating takes extra time and energy and may leave you exhausted.

It often leads to a negative self-fulfilling prophecy: "Because I must succeed to be a worthy person, maybe I'll fail!" Then you do fail! Or: "I'm such a worm for doing poorly! How can a worm like me possibly do well?" Then you can't.

It often alienates others. When they see you constantly rating yourself and putting yourself down, they often lose respect for you, agree with you that you *are* a no-goodnik, and reject you socially or vocationally.

It sometimes leads to grandiosity and overoptimism. "I'm such a great person for doing this project well that now I can do everything well and accomplish anything I want!"

Sarah was almost manic depressive, in that she felt great and noble every time she stuck to her diet for a few weeks—and felt complete self-loathing whenever she went off it. At first, she thought that her constant self-rating was good, because it helped her monitor her eating and kept her no more than twenty pounds "overweight." But she realized, after eight sessions of RET, that she was often seriously depressed, and that even her manic states were bad for her work as an attorney. When manic, she was so elated about her "new" weight that she focused badly on her work and did badly in court and in negotiating for her clients. She forced herself to spend several weeks listing and going over twenty-two serious disadvantages of both "great" and "lousy" self-ratings, got herself into the habit of evaluating only her *dieting* and not *herself*, and became much more stable and productive. As a bonus, she was also able to stick much better to a relatively boring but healthy diet.

Notes to Chapter 14

1. The main books, pamphlets, and cassettes that give details on rational-emotive therapy (RET) techniques are listed and starred in the References at the end of this book. Some of these include: Bernard, 1986, 1991; DiGiuseppe, 1990, 1991; DiMattia & Long, 1990; DiMattia & others, 1987; Dryden, 1990; Dryden & DiGiuseppe, 1990; Dryden & Gordon, 1991; Dryden & Hill, 1992; Ellis, 1957, 1962, 1972a, 1972b, 1973a, 1973b, 1973c, 1974, 1975, 1976, 1977a, 1977b, 1977c, 1978, 1980, 1985a, 1985b, 1988a, 1988b, 1990, 1991a, 1991b, 1991c; Ellis & Becker, 1982; Ellis & DiMattia, 1991; Ellis & Dryden, 1987, 1990, 1991; Ellis & Harper, 1975, 1990; Ellis & Hunter, 1991; Ellis & Knaus, 1977; Ellis, Vega & DiMattia, 1990; Ellis & Velten, 1992; Hauck, 1973, 1974, 1992; Trimpey, 1989; Trimpey & Trimpey, 1990; Velten, 1989; Wolfe, 1980; Wolfe & Brand, 1977; Woods, 1990; Yankura & Dryden, 1990; Young, 1974.

2. Bernard, 1986; Burns, 1980; Ellis, 1973, 1988a; Ellis & Becker, 1982; Ellis & Harper, 1975.

3. Hayakawa, 1962; Johnson, 1946; Korzybski, 1933.

4. Ellis, 1985b, 1988a; Lazarus & Folkman, 1984; Meichenbaum, 1977.

5. Danysh, 1974; Ellis, 1985b, 1988a.

6. Ellis, 1985b, 1988a; Ellis & Hunter, 1991.

7. Bandura, 1986; Ellis & Hunter, 1991.

8. Bourland & Johnston, 1991; Hayakawa, 1962; Johnson, 1946; Korzybski, 1933.

9. Ogles, Lambert, & Craig, 1991; Scogin, Jamison, & Gochneaur, 1989; Starker, 1988.

10. Ellis, McInerney, DiGiuseppe & Yeager, 1988; Ellis & Velten, 1992; Trimpey, 1989; Trimpey & Trimpey, 1990.

11. Ellis, 1976, 1978.

12. Burns, 1980; Dryden, 1990; Dryden & Gordon, 1991; Ellis, 1957, 1962, 1977b, 1988a; A. Ellis & I. Becker, 1982; A. Ellis & R.A. Harper, 1975; Hauck, 1973; Young, 1974.

13. DiGiuseppe, 1990; Ellis, 1974, 1975, 1977c, 1980, 1988b, 1990a; Ellis & Harper, 1990; Knaus, 1975.

14. Ellis, 1985b, 1988a, 1990a.

15. Coué, 1923.

16. Sichel & Ellis, 1984.

17. Ellis, 1985b, 1988a, 1990a; Ellis & Harper, 1975; Jacobson, 1938.

18. Ellis, 1962, 1973, 1985b, 1988a, 1990a; Ellis & Becker, 1982; Ellis & Harper, 1975.

19. Ellis, 1957, 1962, 1985b, 1988a, 1990a.

20. Adler, 1964; Ellis, 1990b; Sampson, 1989.

21. Ellis, 1972b, 1973, 1976b, 1985b, 1988a, 1988b, 1990a, 1991b, 1991c, 1991d, 1992; Ellis & Becker, 1982; Ellis & Dryden, 1987, 1990, 1991; Ellis & Harper, 1975.

15

===

Emotive Ways of Dealing With Your Eating and Other Problems

We have already presented a few emotive techniques of RET to help you deal with your eating and other problems. Now we shall restate some of these and add several more RET emotive-evocative methods.

Rational-Emotive Imagery

Rational-emotive imagery was created by Maxie Maultsby, Jr. in 1971 and can be very helpful in helping you to change your inappropriate feelings about your eating habits or anything else to appropriate ones.[1] To use it, you vividly imagine one of the worst things that might happen to you—such as bingeing and gaining several pounds—and let yourself feel anxious or depressed or be otherwise disturbed about this unfortunate happening. Feel strongly disturbed (C) about this imaginary Activating Event (A) and really, really *feel* it. Then, using the same Activating Event (A), make yourself feel *only* appropriately sorry and disappointed but *not* inappropriately anxious or depressed. Bring about only this *appropriate* negative feeling and make yourself feel it strongly. Repeat this process at least once a day for about thirty days, until you train yourself to semi-automatically feel *appropriately* sorry and disappointed, rather than to feel *in*appropriately anxious, depressed, or self-hating at point C when you vividly visualize—or when you actually experience—an unfortunate Activating Event (at point A). You change C by telling yourself a rational Belief (rB) at point B (your Belief system). Thus, you tell yourself: "It's too bad that A occurred and I don't like it. But there's no reason it *must* not occur, it's not *awful*, and I *can* stand it." Rational-emotive imagery is a self-training or self-conditioning process to make yourself feel appropriately frustrated, sorry, and disappointed rather than inappropriately horrified, self-hating, or enraged when you act poorly or bad events happen to you.[1]

Cindy hated herself because she continually blew her diet, kept gaining rather than losing weight, and carried almost two hundred pounds on her five feet three inches frame. Using rational-emotive imagery, she kept visualizing the worst: that she steadily continued to go off her diet and kept creeping up to 200, 210, 220 pounds. Imagining this, she felt very depressed and almost suicidal. Working on her feelings, she made herself feel, instead, only sorry and disappointed about her *behavior*, but not horrified about her rotten *self*. How? By telling herself, "I really hate my overeating and my putting myself down for it. But although they, these actions, are quite bad, I am definitely not a *crummy person*. Just a person who acts crummily in this important area. And one who *can* change!" After using rational-emotive imagery (REI) for thirty days, at least once a day, she trained herself to feel automatically sorry and disappointed, rather than depressed, about her weight. Then she had a much easier time dieting.

Shame-Attacking Exercises

Albert Ellis realized, in the 1950s, that shame and guilt are the essence of much human disturbance. In the

1960s he invented the now famous RET shame-attacking exercises.[2] Whenever you are afflicted—or, rather, afflict yourself—with feelings of shame, embarrassment, humiliation, or guilt, you are almost always telling yourself a rational Belief (rB), such as, "I don't like acting this way, and I dislike others putting me down for behaving the way I do." You then feel sorry and regretful but *not* ashamed. But you also are adding an irrational Belief (iB) like: "I *must not* act this shameful way! It's *awful* if people dislike me for it! I'm an *incompetent, rotten person!*" *Then* you feel ashamed.

Using RET, you do not Dispute (D) why your act was foolish and why people dislike you for it because these facts may be valid. But you do Dispute your irrational Beliefs and change them back to rational preferences, such as, "Acting this way is undesirable, but there's no reason why I *must* not act undesirably, why it's *awful* if I do and if people dislike me for it, and why my act makes me an *incompetent, rotten person.*"

Fine, but RET is emotive and behavioral, as well as cognitive. So to do its shame-attacking exercises, you deliberately, consciously do something you personally consider "shameful" or "humiliating" and you do it while working on yourself to *not* feel ashamed. What kind of shame-attacking things do you do? Well, first of all, nothing that would harm someone else—such as slapping someone in the face. And nothing that would get you into trouble—such as walking naked in public or telling your boss that he or she is a louse.

Pick something practical as a shame-attacking exercise. For example, wearing an outfit that you think is attractive but not exactly in style. Or refusing to tip a waiter who has given poor service.

Or pick something downright foolish—such as yelling out the time or singing aloud on the street; or asking for a toothbrush in a clothing store; or telling someone you just got out of a mental hospital; or asking a stranger for a date;

or wearing clothes that show rather than conceal that you are too fat or too thin.

Make sure, however, that as you do this "shameful" act, you work hard at what you tell yourself *not* to feel ashamed or embarrassed. And preferably do this and other supposedly "shameful" acts many times, until you show yourself that although many of your performances are socially wrong or foolish, none of them are humiliating, and none make you a *terrible person*. Only you do!

Marvin was thoroughly ashamed to be seen in a bathing suit because he felt that he was far "too fat," especially around the middle. So he never went to beaches and pools, although he loved swimming. He Disputed his irrational Beliefs, "I'm a thorough slob if people see how fat I really am! My stomach is revolting and shameful!"

He felt better, but still didn't do any swimming. So he and his therapist worked out a shame-attacking exercise in which he went to lectures and deliberately asked foolish questions and thereby made himself the laughing stock of large audiences. For example, after a lecturer had presented many facts to highlight his claim that many people were needlessly hostile, Marvin would get up and ask, "Do you really have any facts about people's hostility? Do you really think that some individuals *are* that way?"

Marvin did this shame-attacking exercise a dozen times, got laughed at each time, but soon felt no shame. Getting used to acting foolishly and being laughed at, he was able to follow up with lying on crowded beaches and going swimming in a scanty bathing suit. Being unashamed, but still disliking his appearance, he was motivated to diet and exercise and acquire a much more athletic-looking, though hardly really thin and stomachless, body.

Forceful Coping Statements

Use the same kind of coping self-statements we talked about in the previous chapter and say them to yourself

many times very forcefully, until you really believe them.[3]
For example:

"Yes, I weigh much more than I would like to weigh.
But that never makes me a HOPELESSLY FAT,
AWFUL PERSON!"

"I would very much LIKE to be thinner but I NEV-
ER HAVE TO BE!"

"People often unfairly put me down about my weight
and other things. I dislike their unfairness but they
SHOULD, DEFINITELY SHOULD be that way
right now. For that's the way THEY BEHAVE at
present."

"Having people's approval is great. But I CER-
TAINLY NEVER NEED IT! I *CAN* be happy without it!"

Forceful Self-Disputing

RET therapists recognized, a number of years ago,
that people often do their Disputing of their irrational
Beliefs lightly and unconvincingly and that they had better
do so more forcefully and vigorously. Several methods of
forceful self-disputing were therefore created, which you
can use to debate your own irrationalities.[4]

Taped disputing. You can talk to a tape recorder and
state one of your main irrational Beliefs (iBs), such as,
"Whenever I gain a few pounds I am proving that I am
completely undisciplined, am hopeless, and am no
damned good for being such a jerk!" You then vigorously
Dispute this iB on the tape and listen to it later. Get some
friends and associates to listen to it, to see if your Disputing was really quite vigorous and convincing. If not, continue this taped Disputing until you forcefully convince
yourself that your iB is false and self-defeating.

Role-play disputing. You can let one of your friends or

associates rigidly and powerfully present and hold on to one (or more) of your irrational Beliefs (iBs). Then you try to vigorously talk them out of these iBs.

You can also uphold this iB yourself and have one or more of your friends vehemently try to talk you out of it. You then can learn some strong Disputes that you might not figure out for yourself.

Sandra used forceful self-disputing when she had trouble finishing her course as a body trainer because she was (she thought) thirty pounds overweight when all the other women in her class seemed to have almost perfect, as well as firm and muscular, figures. She failed to stop her abysmal self-castigation with RET Disputing, largely because she didn't Dispute very vigorously.

So she put on tape some of her irrational Beliefs (iBs), such as, "I hate my fat ass and thighs and *can't stand* my classmates seeing them. I'm a gross, blubbery slob compared to all the other women in my class and I should be a washer woman instead of a body trainer!" She vigorously contradicted these Beliefs on a cassette tape and played this Disputing tape to some of her friends. As a shame-attacking exercise she even played it to two of the women in her class, listened to everyone's critique, did her tape over in a stronger Disputing manner, and finally accepted herself with her "fat" figure and went on to be a successful, though still "fat-of-ass," body trainer.

Use of Humor

When people are emotionally upset, they often hang on to their irrational Beliefs overseriously and unhumorously. RET therefore teaches them to laugh, not at themselves, but at their self- defeating ideas, to take them to absurd extremes and to show how funny and contradictory they often are.[5] You can look for the humorous side of your destructive notions and can wittily rip them up.

For example, it is ironic and funny that you think you can change other people's negative views of your weight, which is often untrue, and that you can't change your own denouncing yourself for being overweight or underweight—which, of course, you can! And it is outrageously funny that you think that no one will love you when you are, say, twenty pounds "too fat" when, actually, some people will only be attracted to you *because* you have those twenty "extra" pounds.

RET also uses rational humorous songs to help people laugh at their overly serious, destructive Beliefs. At the Institute for Rational-Emotive Therapy in New York, we give all our clinic clients a song sheet, so that they can sing an antidepression song to themselves when they are depressed, sing an anti-anxiety song when they are anxious, and sing other rational humorous songs when they feel disturbed. We find that they often use these songs beneficially.

Here are some typical rational humorous songs that you can use when you are disturbed about your weight problems or almost anything else:

I'M DEPRESSED, DEPRESSED!
(TUNE: *THE BAND PLAYED ON* BY CHARLES B. WARD)

Whenever my weight's in a mild fatty state,
I'm depressed, depressed!
Whenever I'm stricken with thickening weight,
I feel most distressed!
When I am not fated to be slender stated,
I can't tolerate it at all!
Whenever my weight's in a mild fatty state,
I just bawl, bawl, bawl!

WHINE, WHINE, WHINE
(TUNE: *YALE WHIFFENPOOF SONG*, BY GUY SCULL—
A HARVARD MAN!)

I cannot have all of my fatness killed—
Whine, whine, whine!

I cannot change all of my body build—
Whine, whine, whine!
Life really owes me the thinness I miss,
Fate has to grant me real skinny bliss!
And since I must suffer far more than this—
Whine, whine, whine!

PERFECT RATIONALITY
(Tune: *Funiculi, Funicula* by Luigi Denza)

Some think the world must have a right direction,
And so do I! And so do I!
Some think that, with the slightest imperfection,
They can't get by—and so do I!
For I, I have to prove I'm superhuman,
And better far than people are!
To show I have miraculous acumen—
And always rate among the Great

Perfect, perfect rationality
Is, of course, the only thing for me!
How can I ever think of being
If I must live fallibly?
Rationality must be a perfect thing for me!

LOVE ME, LOVE ME, ONLY ME!
(Tune: *Yankee Doodle Dandy*)

Love me, love me, only me
Or I'll die without you!
Make your love a guarantee,
So I can never doubt you!
Love me, love me totally—really, really try, dear,
But if you demand love, too,
I'll hate you till I die, dear!

Love me, love me all the time,
Thoroughly and wholly!

Love turns into slushy slime
Less you love me solely!
Love me with great tenderness,
With no ifs or buts, dear.
If you love me somewhat less,
I'll hate your goddamned guts, dear!

YOU FOR ME AND ME FOR ME
(TUNE: *TEA FOR TWO* BY VINCENT YOUMANS)

Picture you upon my knee,
Just you for me, and me for me!
And then you'll see
How happy I will be, dear!
Though you beseech me
You never will reach me—
For I am autistic as any real mystic,
And only relate to myself with a great to-do, dear!
If you dare to try to care
You'll see my caring soon will wear,
For I can't pair and make our sharing fair!
If you want a family
We'll both agree you'll baby me—
Then you'll see how happy I will be!

I WISH I WERE NOT CRAZY
(TUNE: *DIXIE* BY DAN EMMETT)

Oh, I wish I were really put together—
Smooth and fine as patent leather!
Oh, how great to be rated innately sedate!
But I'm afraid that I was fated
To be rather aberrated—
Oh, how sad to be mad as my Mom and my Dad!

Oh, I wish I were not crazy! Hooray, hooray!
I wish my mind were less inclined
To be the kind that's hazy!

I could agree to really be less crazy,
But I, alas, am just too goddamned lazy!

(Lyrics by Albert Ellis, Copyright 1977 to 1991 by
    Institute for Rational-Emotive Therapy)

Relationship Methods

RET teaches people that they do not absolutely need others' love and approval in order to accept themselves but that it can significantly add to their lives and sometimes, if it is given unconditionally, help them to fully accept themselves. Self-acceptance, as shown throughout this book, is most helpful and you can always decide—yes, decide—to give it to yourself.[6] Relationships with others are also most important and beneficial to people with weight and other problems.

You can also seek out some friends and relatives who will unconditionally accept you; and a good therapist, especially an RET practitioner, can prove very helpful in that respect. Group therapy and self-help groups, if available in your community, can provide support and the possibility of finding good relationships. The more, however, you learn RET, and unconditionally accept yourself and others, the better family, mating, and social relationships you are likely to make. Unconditional love frequently begets return love!

Gerard was sure that all attractive women disapproved of him because he was six feet four inches tall and very thin, because he wore thick ugly glasses, and because he was a government employee and made less money than other accountants. He made himself so defensive and angry that most women he met were turned off by his hostile manner and believed, rightly, that he would treat them shabbily. In RET group therapy he was helped to give up his anger against women and feel only appropriately frustrated and sorry when they rejected intimacies with him.

By getting himself to unconditionally accept women he found that most of them had serious problems of their own. So, although not trained in psychology, he used RET with them, showed real interest in their troubles, and was quite helpful to several of them. Seeing that he was uniquely accepting of them and of himself, some of his dates became attached to him in spite of his looks, and some of his handsome male friends were astounded by, and envious of, how women found him so sexually attractive. When he finally married a remarkably bright and good-looking woman, these male friends were happy to be free of his competition!

Notes to Chapter 15

1. Maultsby, 1971; Maultsby & Ellis, 1974.

2. Ellis, 1969, 1973a, 1985b, 1988a, 1990a; Ellis & Abrahms, 1978; Ellis & Becker, 1982; Ellis & Dryden, 1987; Ellis & Harper, 1975.

3. Ellis, 1975, 1988a, 1990a; Ellis & Abrahms, 1978; Ellis & Dryden, 1987, 1990, 1991.

4. Ellis, 1988a, 1990a; Ellis & Abrahms, 1978; Ellis & Dryden, 1991.

5. Ellis, 1977a, 1977c, 1977d, 1987b, 1990a.

6. Ellis, 1957, 1971, 1977a, 1979, 1982, 1986, 1988a, 1990a, 1990c, 1991a, 1991d, 1991f; Ellis & Becker, 1982; Ellis & Dryden, 1991; Ellis & Harper, 1961, 1975.

16

Behavioral Ways of Dealing With Your Eating and Other Problems

We have mentioned several behavioral methods of RET that you can use to help overcome your eating problems, the emotional difficulties that often accompany them, and other disturbances that you may help create. We shall now summarize and expand on these techniques.

Behavioral Desensitization

RET specializes in behavioral desensitization—especially in showing people how to bite the bullet of their irrational fears and desensitize themselves *in vivo*, or in the course of live action.[1] Thus, if you are afraid of elevators, public speaking, gourmet restaurants, or almost anything else, you can deliberately force yourself, many times, to confront these "dangerous" pursuits until you overcome your irrational fears and learn how to handle yourself when you confront these dangers.

Watch it, however, because some of your eating fears may be pretty rational. Your fear of gourmet restaurants may be legitimate in the sense that the food will be so tempting that you may well eat more of it—or eat more of the wrong delicious food. As we show later in this chapter, stimulus control, or staying away from tempting situations, is often the better part of valor.

But elevators, trains, and planes are ordinarily *not* fearful; and if you make them "frightening" by telling yourself that going in them *must* at all times be one hundred percent safe and comfortable, you will create an irrational fear—or panic state—that may greatly encourage you to overeat, to drink, to resort to drugs, or to do some other foolish acts to temporarily calm yourself. In such cases, use RET to convince yourself that you don't *need* one hundred percent safety and comfort—ninety-eight percent is good enough!—and PYA (push your ass) to do the "fearful" thing many times, until you cognitive-behaviorally conquer it!

The same with "frightening" or "horrible" foods. If lettuce or some other food is excellent for your diet but you are phobic about it and practically vomit at the thought of eating it, strongly convince yourself that eating it is, at the worst, *unpleasant* and *uncomfortable*, but hardly *awful* or *gravesome*; and force yourself, perhaps with delicious dressing, to eat and eat it, until you topple your phobia. A word of caution, again: *Don't* try to overcome your genuine allergies to certain foods—such as, perhaps, milk products. *Do* counterattack, with words and actions, your self-defeating food phobias.

Timothy was phobic about eating solid foods, especially steak, because he had once severely choked while gobbling down a large hunk of sirloin. He only ate mushy and liquid foods, and was thoroughly ashamed of himself for avoiding all weightier fare.

Using RET, Timothy first forgave himself for his food phobias by Disputing his irrational Beliefs, "I must not have any silly phobia like this. I'm perfectly able to ingest rough food and must not stick to baby foods, like I childishly do!"

Once he stopped putting himself down for his food phobia, Timothy still had the problem of overcoming it. Seeing that two of his friends tried RET to overcome their public speaking and train riding phobias, he decided to try the same kind of *in vivo* desensitization that they had successfully employed. So he forced himself, at least once a day, to eat very solid foods like toast and steak, despite his great discomfort and his fear of choking to death, Timothy persisted, and within a month was eating much more solid than mushy food. And whenever he temporarily fell back to his phobic eating he still steadfastly accepted himself and returned to his more solid and "dangerous" diet again.

Staying With Discomfort

As we stress throughout this book, low frustration tolerance (LFT) or discomfort disturbance (DD) lurks behind many eating (and other) disorders.[2] Take Myra, for example. She first made herself terribly anxious about looking for office temp jobs because she told herself it wasn't only hard but *too* hard calling the agencies, going for interviews, working with new people, not getting health benefits, etc. Second, she kept eating bagels, while working on her coffee breaks, because it was *too hard* to bear her discomfort anxiety about working. Third, she kept breaking her Weight Watcher's diet because it was *too hard* to stay on it. Fourth, she often purged because it was *too hard* to go back to her dieting. Fifth, she refused to work at her RET group therapy and to do her RET homework because it was *too hard* to keep filling out the self-help report forms and to do rational-emotive imagery that she had agreed with the group to do. So she insisted on destructively downing herself for her LFT. Sixth, she prematurely quit therapy because it was *too hard* to pay the moderate fee the Institute for Rational-Emotive Therapy charged her for being a member of the group. LFT all the way! Not to mention *indulgence* in self-downing. When, after returning to group, she finally worked hard on her self-flagellation and for the first time in her life began to accept herself *with* her LFT, she found it much easier—though never completely easy and enjoyable—to tackle her work and her compulsive bagel eating.

When you are in a really rotten situation—such as a boring job or marriage—RET often recommends that you *not* cop out too quickly and arrange for a better set of conditions. Instead, if you are afflicted with low frustration tolerance, you can choose to deliberately stay in the poor situation and use RET to *refuse* to upset yourself about it. Thus, you can surrender your rage, depression, or panic *about* what is unfortunately happening and *then* decide what action, if any, you'd better take.[3] Forcing yourself, in this manner, to temporarily stay frustrated, may well help you improve your LFT, give you more time to plan what to do, and improve your decision making. As you temporarily *accept* your poor job, home, or social conditions you will be less likely to drive yourself to undereat or to overeat to "deal" with them.

THE CASE OF CYNTHIA

Cynthia absolutely couldn't stand her boss and her co-worker, George, who got along beautifully with this boss and was unfairly favored over Cynthia. So, in the course of a year, Cynthia gained twenty-five pounds, mainly by having a few Martinis every lunch time so that she could get through the afternoon without killing someone. Several members of Cynthia's therapy group kept urging her to quit her job, even though she would get a vested interest in a pension fund if she stayed for another eleven months. "It isn't worth it!" said one of the group members. "If you wait the eleven months you'll give yourself an ulcer—and hell knows what else!"

Cynthia was all set to quit when one of the older group members, Gregory, spoke up. "I can well understand what you're going through and I truly sympathize with you. But let me tell you what happened to me when I was in a very similar position three years ago. My boss and my supervisor were both giving me a hard time and were favoring a muddle-headed but very attractive woman colleague who may well have been sleeping with both of them. Maybe not, since she was too stupid even to be good in bed!

"Anyway, I did quit, just as you're about to do, and lost some profit-sharing rights I would have obtained had I stayed a year longer. So you can see the similarities between your position and mine!

"So I quit. In a rage. It took me a whole year to get another good position, since, to say the least, I got lukewarm recommendations when new employers called my boss or supervisor. When I finally got a job, which I took in desperation, my supervisor again unfairly favored my office partner, probably because they had been friends for a long time, and I couldn't get anywhere. Naturally, because I took my rage with me, I seethed—just like you began overeating—to calm myself, and worked very badly.

"This time, however, I joined this RET group, decided to work on myself, gave up my anger, forgave my unfair supervisor, and now she actually favors me over my colleague. So don't cop out. Work on *you*. Stay on this job till *you* stop raging. Then if you want to quit, quit—and take your unangry self to the next job."

Cynthia listened to Gregory rather than to the other group members, *un*angrily stayed on her job for another year, and then, as conditions at work were still stacked against her, she left for another difficult position which she was well able to handle. Meanwhile, she stopped her drinking at lunch and lost fifteen pounds.

Paradoxical Homework

Many people who resist changing their destructive thoughts, feelings, and actions are able to do so by paradoxically acting against them.[4] Thus, if you think you are too fat or too thin to make dates with people you find suitable and you are terrified of rejection, deliberately go to social gatherings and make sure that you get rejected at least five times every week. In doing so, you'll almost certainly get some acceptance—and you'll see that you probably won't die of the many rejections you get.

Marsha found that whenever she ate peanuts she finished the whole jar. So she paradoxically forced herself, several times, to finish five or six jars of peanuts, until she became revolted with them. Thereafter, she rarely ate any peanuts or, if she did, only ate a few of them.

Reinforcement Methods

Because overeating—and, at times, starvation—is so reinforcing to many people, they had better pleasantly reinforce themselves whenever they eat properly. Also, because people with eating disorders have, as we show in this book, various emotional problems that contribute to their self-defeating eating, and because they frequently won't do their cognitive, emotive, and behavioral homework to help overcome their disturbances, they had better often reinforce themselves for doing this homework.[5]

To use reinforcement methods, you find some activities—such as reading, watching TV, exercising, socializing, or even eating certain special foods—and you do them only *after* you have done some activities you avoid, such as dieting, working at RET Disputing, or attending self-help meetings. Remember: *Only* reinforce or reward yourself *after* you do beneficial acts that you often refuse to do.

Paul rewarded himself with a quarter of a pint of ice cream every Sunday only after he had stayed with his low-fat, low-salt diet all week. Mabel did her evening telephone socializing only after she stayed away from all alcohol each day. Bobbye allowed herself to run for three miles three times every week only if she did ten minutes of RET Disputing every day.

Penalty Methods

People with long-term eating problems, and especially those who have emotional disturbances contributing to these problems, are often not very reinforceable, because they receive so much pleasure or relief from their eating and from their temporarily allaying their disturbed feelings while eating that all other kinds of reinforcements are too bland and pale to be effective.[6] If you find that reinforcements do not work for you, try some stiff penalties! Every time, for example, that you overeat, or starve yourself to achieve perfect thinness, or purge after bingeing, make yourself quickly eat something very obnoxious, burn a hundred dollar bill, have sex with someone you loathe, or do some other *really* offensive thing. Yes, *really* offensive!

Josephine binged and purged two or three times a week but stopped completely after she penalized herself by going to bed with her ex-husband, whom she loathed, quickly after each bingeing session. Mohammed burned a dollar bill for every calorie he ate more than 1,200 a day. Within two weeks, he had burned $502.00 and he started keeping to his 1,200 a day limit. Sylvia ate a pound of turnips, which she thoroughly hated, every time she ate any cookies, and within two months, was eating no cookies.

As you use penalties like these for your bad eating or other habits, make sure that you do not damn yourself along with your self-penalizing. This will only make you feel like a *hopeless, rotten person* and will most likely increase your disturbance and dysfunctional behavior.

Relapse Prevention

As we have kept noting in this book, strict dieters, especially "overeaters" who are trying to lose weight, relapse in about ninety-five percent of the cases and gain back their lost pounds—and more! RET, following Alan Marlatt and other behavior therapists, has adopted some useful relapse prevention methods.[7] You can use these as follows:

Cognitively, you can look at your irrational Beliefs (iBs) that drive you to relapse, such as "I *can't stand* not eating this delicious food!" "I'll go crazy if I keep on this diet!" "I'm an inadequate person because I have to keep dieting forever!" Look for these iBs, preferably *before* you relapse, and forcefully Dispute them.

Emotively, use rational-emotive imagery to imagine you are really being tempted to go off your diet, let yourself feel anxious or depressed about this image, work on changing your feeling to one of disappointment and regret, and see yourself as resisting temptation.

Behaviorally, stay away from places and people that are likely to tempt you to relapse. Use stimulus control to make desirable food that leads to undesirable results out of reach.[8]

Maria relapsed so many times on her diet when she went out to lunch that she made her own lunch and ate it in the office. Jonathan only had a charge account at a health food shop and kept away from all other kinds of shops and restaurants.

Stimulus Control

As mentioned above, stimulus control is often an excellent behavioral method of staying away from unhealthy food, liquor, love slobbism, and other disturbed indulgences and is often used in RET.[9] Thus, you can stay out of restaurants and bars, keep no self-sabotaging food in your house, stay away from "friends" who keep urging you to eat or do other foolish things, carry with you very little money and no checks, credit cards, or charge account numbers, turn off your stove, etc.

Marlena bought no food during the day and only carried around her two small apples. Billy never went out to eat with friends and only served them healthy, non-fattening foods when he invited them to his apartment. Karen limited her total food purchases to a small amount every week and refused all food that was offered to her by others. Samuel, who hated to cook and prepare food, only ate at home. Josef only ate out at an eaterie that served poor food and that he had to walk three miles to get to.

Skill Training

People are often disturbed because they lack important skills—such as assertiveness or social skills—and they also lack these skills because they are disturbed: for example, have a dire need of approval and a horror of rejection. RET, therefore, helps them to change their irrational Beliefs (iBs) and their emotional Consequences (Cs) that often lead to their lack of important skills; and it also, if required, teaches how to go back to the Activating Events (A's) in their lives and to acquire better skills.[9]

Thus, if you are socially unskilled, and therefore upset and overeating, you can change your irrational Beliefs (iBs) about your lack of skills, about your upsetness, and about your overeating. You can convince yourself that you are *not* a worm for being unskilled, that you *can* stand your upsetness without temporarily drowning it in overeating, and that you are *not a thoroughly rotten weakling* for indulging in food. As you do this, you can read, take courses, get a mentor, join a group, go for therapy, and otherwise *learn* better social skills. If you really want to diet but don't have the skills required for doing so properly, you can learn and practice shopping, cooking, calorie counting, and other diet-related skills.

Bettyann first stopped damning herself for her bingeing and purging, started attending Weight Watchers regularly, and became so good at proper food selection that she began to help several of her friends with their eating. Harvey worked on his dire need for women's approval, gained social skills by forcing himself to date many women and learn by his mistakes, and thereby rid himself of his severe depression. Then he no longer stuffed himself (though already five feet six inches tall and 210 pounds) to partially alleviate his depressed state.

Notes to Chapter 16

1. Ellis, 1962, 1973, 1985, 1990a; Ellis & Abrahms, 1978; Ellis & Dryden, 1987, 1990, 1991; Ellis & Whiteley, 1979.

2. Ellis, 1957, 1962, 1987a, 1991c, 1991d; Ellis & Becker, 1982; Ellis & Dryden, 1987, 1990, 1991; Ellis, Vega, & DiMattia, 1990; Ellis & Whiteley, 1979.

3. Ellis, 1962, 1985, 1988a; Ellis & Dryden, 1990; Ellis & Grieger, 1977, 1986; Hauck, 1974.

4. Ellis, 1985b, 1988a, 1990a; Ellis & Abrahms, 1978; Frankl, 1959.

5. Ellis, 1985b, 1990a; Ellis & Abrams, 1978; Ellis & Dryden, 1987, 1991; Ellis & Whiteley, 1979.

6. Ellis, 1985b, 1988a, 1990a; Ellis & Abrams, 1978; Ellis & Velten, 1992; Ellis & Whiteley, 1979.

7. Ellis, 1985b, 1988a, 1990a; Ellis & Velten, 1992; Marlatt & Gordon, 1985.

8. Ellis, 1985b, 1988a; Ellis & Velten, 1992.

9. Ellis, 1972e, 1990; Ellis & Abrahms, 1978; Ellis & Dryden, 1991; Ellis & Whiteley, 1978.

17

Some Tentative Conclusions

Much is now known about weight loss and eating disorders, but much still remains to be discovered. So let us make some tentative—and presumably rational—conclusions about the research findings we report in this book and about the clinical findings from our own combined clinical practice specializing in treating people with eating problems and other emotional difficulties for over 75 years.

First, let us address readers who are sure that they are "overweight." Watch it! Don't cavalierly decide that you are "fat" because you are ten or twenty pounds over the "norm" of our culture. If you are fifty or more pounds "overweight" take care and talk to your regular physician about this. See if you have any special problems—such as thyroid or metabolism deficiencies—and do your best to correct them. Try dieting, if you will, but only under the guidance of a good internist, endocrinologist, or other physician. Only with her or his help consider any fluid, "miraculous," "unique," or "special" diet.

If you are "moderately" overweight and this kind of "fatness" tends to exist in several close members of your family, seriously consider staying pretty much the way you are. There is a good chance that your natural biological setpoint—or "normal" weight for you as an individual—is pretty well fixed and that only with continual rigorous dieting—yes, for the rest of your life—will you be able to make and keep yourself "thin." You can try reducing, of course, but most likely you will have real trouble and may easily fail—and fail and fail! You will very probably lose and gain—l-o-s-e and GAIN!— fifteen or twenty pounds for the rest of your life. Which is quite unhealthy; and isn't worth it. Well, *is* it?

If your biological setpoint is fairly high, moreover, and you nevertheless *do* consistently stay fifteen or more pounds below it, you will probably steadily feel starved and preoccupied with food and will spend so much time and energy keeping "slim" that you'd better keep asking yourself, "Is this *really* worth it? *Must* I always be as thin as I *want* to be? Or do I have better alternatives?"

For, you almost always do have other good choices if your setpoint is high and consistently trying to be "thin" is going to give you a lifetime of real trouble. You can refuse to take your "fatness"-hating relatives and friends too seriously. You can find lovers and mates who genuinely accept and like your body even though you are "overweight." You can make real efforts to consistently have a *healthy* rather than a *"thin"* constitution. You can work at achieving one of the main goals stressed in this book: Fully and *un*conditionally accepting yourself although you—and some of your friends and relatives—think that you are distinctly above the "ideal" weight.

So keep in mind: You never *have to* be "thin," even though you would *prefer* to be. You can have your *desire* to shed fifteen or twenty pounds and to keep it off forever, and stubbornly refuse to make it into a *necessity.* Your being "overweight" in our society may have real disadvantages, but your forcing yourself to be always thin may create many more pains and hazards. Carefully weigh the consequences of *both* choices!

If you do decide that you really want to be "thin"—or even just "thinner"—try to make sure that you don't have an eating disorder, such as bulimia or anorexia. When you are bulimic you will keep your weight down, all right, but mainly by bingeing and vomiting. This is an emotional and behavioral disturbance, as we point out in chapter 11, and is related to self-downing and low frustration tolerance. If you are a binger and a regurgitator carefully read chapter 11 and make sure that you get medical and psychological help. This kind of eating disorder is a *real* problem. Run, don't walk, to the nearest good doctor and rational-emotive or cognitive-behavioral therapist!

Similarly with anorexia nervosa. As we also show in chapter 11, anorectics practically always have serious emotional problems, including perfectionism, obsessive-compulsions, and self-hatred. They often make themselves pathologically thin, destroy their bodies, and not infrequently die of starvation. If you suspect that you are even moderately anorectic make a beeline for medical and psychological treatment. No excuse, now. Go!

What about dieting for the sake of your physical and emotional health? By all means take this approach. As many recent nutritional, medical, and psychological studies have shown, your carefully selecting the food that you eat, your ingesting the right kinds of vitamins and minerals (especially by eating a variety of healthy goods), and your properly (and not obsessively-compulsively) exercising will almost certainly aid your health and longevity. And often also help you emotionally! This is notably true when you have special physical problems (such as diabetes) and when you are allergic to certain substances or have biochemical deficiencies that require special food, vitamins, or other nutritional procedures.

So good eating and exercising are very important to health and happy living. Unfortunately, most people—and that can easily include *you*—are prone to low frustration tolerance, to indulgence in immediate gratification, to procrastination, and to other self-defeating ways of thinking, feeling, and behaving with which they often sabotage their acquiring and maintaining good eating and exercising habits. If you, like the great majority of people, have considerable low frustration tolerance (otherwise known as short-range hedonism), and if you also tend to berate and damn yourself as a person for being lax in this respect (and thereby *increase* your emotional difficulties), seriously review the parts of this book, particularly chapters 14, 15, and 16, that show you many rational-emotive and cognitive-behavioral methods you can use to deal with these emotional problems. Also, read and listen to some of the materials in the References at the end of this book that are mainly on rational-emotive therapy (RET). These are preceded by an asterisk (*) and will not cure you of all your emotional, food-related problems, but they certainly may help.

Let us conclude by reminding you of three major insights of RET, particularly as they apply to rational eating:

Insight No. 1: As a human, you are born with a strong healthy tendency to think, to think about your thinking, and to think about your thoughts, your feelings, and your behaviors. You therefore almost always have the ability to create good eating (and noneating) habits and to change them when they are self-destructive. But, being a highly fallible human, you are born and reared with strong physical and psychological tendencies to think and act unwholesomely and self-destructively and to create needless problems for yourself and others. This is particularly true in regard to eating, a vitally important area of life in which you *easily* can choose to eat badly and destructively. Yes, *easily*. Yes, *choose*. For, as long as you have plenty of food around, which most of us who live in Western civilization do have, from childhood onward you can largely choose to eat or to refuse to eat and can choose to have healthy or unhealthy thoughts and feelings about eating and dieting. Although you largely learn from your parents and your culture to eat "good" and to avoid "bad" foods, you personally *decide*, even at an early age, to eat too much or too little, as well as to eat in a self-helping or self-sabotaging manner. When you pick destructive food habits and when you stubbornly persist at them in spite of your knowing that they are destructive, you largely do so for the same reason that you act neurotically in other areas of your life: You take your preferences for and against certain foods and you make them—oh, yes, MAKE them—into arrogant, absolutist demands.

Thus, when you create neurotic, destructive food habits, you take your self-helping, preferential beliefs— such as, "I *like* ice cream and strawberry shortcake very much BUT they contain too much fat and sugar, so I'll only eat small portions of them and keep myself healthy even though this is frustrating"—and make these into dysfunctional, musturbatory beliefs—such as, "Because I like ice cream and strawberry shortcake very much, I *absolutely must* keep eating large portions of them. It's *awful* if I frustrate myself by refraining from eating them! I *can't stand* this kind of frustration and my life is *terrible* if I continually refrain!"

Insight No. 1 of RET, in other words, holds that food and your wishes and antipathies about it do not directly cause your neurotic behavior of eating too much or too little. Instead, you almost always can *choose* to think rationally or irrationally and to feel appropriately or inappropriately about food, and by your *self*-created beliefs and feelings, consciously or unconsciously *select* your self-helping or self-defeating eating habits. As that great American philosopher Pogo said: In regard to our neurotic food (and other) actions, "we have met the enemy—and it is us!"

Insight No. 2 of RET holds that the main reason why

you still defeat yourself in regard to eating today is not because you *once* did so in your childhood or adolescence and because your old thinking and emotional, and behavioral habits *just* linger on. No. That's what the Freudians and Orthodox Behaviorists say, but not what RET assumes. Instead, RET holds that your old neurotic ideas and feelings remain alive today because you *actively keep constructing and reconstructing them* when faced with current food (and other) stimuli. Thus, you originally built (usually during childhood) a *general philosophy* of low frustration tolerance, such as, "Whenever I strongly desire anything, such as ice cream and strawberry shortcake, I *absolutely must not* be frustrated; and it's *awful* and I *can't stand* it when I am. Therefore, I *need* what I *strongly want* right now, even though I may later suffer from indulging in it."

Insight No. 2 says that your irrational Belief (iB), and the powerful feeling of low frustration tolerance (neediness instead of wantingness) that goes with it, are both consciously and unconsciously *repeated* and *re-experienced* many, many times by you over the years. And today when having the Activating Event (A) of available ice cream and strawberry shortcake presented to you, and also having the knowledge that it is unhealthy for you to eat much of this "treat," you *still* Believe (B) and actively repeat to yourself, what we noted a few paragraphs back, "Because I like this food very much, I *absolutely must* keeping eating large portions of it. It's *awful* and I *can't stand* frustrating myself by refraining from eating it!" *Insight No. 2*, then, states that it is not your *past* history or philosophy that drives you to act neurotically about eating harmful food today. Rather, it is your *present* (conscious and unconscious) *reiteration* of that basic or core philosophy (sometimes called a schema) that neurotically moves you. So, whatever your history, you'd better *now* make yourself aware of this core philosophy and how it affects your eating and *now* determine to drastically and powerfully change it.

Insight No. 3 of RET holds that if you have constructed and persisted at maintaining your self-defeating, neurotic eating behavior it will almost always be quite difficult for you to change it to self-helping thoughts, feelings, and actions—and to keep it changed. Why? For several reasons:

1. Your desires for harmful food (such as ice cream and strawberry shortcake) and your aversions for proper eating (such as consistent dieting) are often biologically based and are also learned during your early life. You have *practiced* indulging in them for many years and have *made them* strong and powerful.

2. Your tendency to have considerable low frustration tolerance about eating (and other pleasures and aversions) also has biological roots. Practically all humans *easily* go for immediate gratification instead of future gain and therefore often indulge in harmful pursuits (such as overeating or overspending) instead of disciplining themselves to achieve more lasting pleasures (such as healthy bodies and useful savings). Therefore, you (and many other people) can naturally and effortlessly acquire undisciplined eating habits. Most children are also indulged during their early years with immediate gratifications and consequently also *acquire* considerable low frustration tolerance.

3. Humans, as RET has shown since the early 1960s, have no trouble thinking unrealistically and illogically and therefore quickly jumping from preferential, rational Beliefs (rBs)—such as "I greatly *like* fattening foods"—to musturbatory irrational Beliefs (iBs)—such as, "No matter what the ultimate Consequences (Cs), I *absolutely must have* the foods I like." Along with their innately propended iBs, nearly all people, especially when they are young, often give priority to their feelings even when these lead to poor results. For example, "I know that fattening foods are bad for me, but I *greatly feel* like eating them right now. So to hell with my self-discipline!" Both cognitively and emotionally, then, you (like other people) are innately

prone to create and go along with self-destructive food habits.

4. Like most humans, you are probably genetically prone to have setpoints and metabolism factors that make it very hard for you to lose and keep off "extra" weight; and some of you may even have setpoints that make it almost impossible for you to gain desired weight. In either case, disciplined eating may not get you to achieve and keep you at the weight or figure you distinctly prefer.

5. When you have destructive thoughts, feelings, and behaviors in regard to eating (or almost anything else), you have usually practiced and practiced them for a number of years—often from childhood till today. So you have, first, been born with a strong tendency (as virtually all humans are) to *habituate* yourself to pronounced actions (like eating) and inactions (like refraining from exercise). Habit-making is the natural, biological human tendency. Habit-breaking is also biologically possible—but much more difficult to achieve!

Second, whatever eating and non-eating you have developed, including destructive ones you have practiced and practiced over the years, and thereby reinforced and solidified them, you probably did not consciously *notice* the activity you used to maintain these habits. Thus, you rarely noticed your active thoughts, "That strawberry shortcake looks great! I must buy it. It's a pleasure to carry it home. Eating a portion of it is fine! Putting the rest of it away is too frustrating! I'll only take a little bit more. No, I really have to finish it. I promise myself that I won't buy another cake—tomorrow!" But, notice it or not, you *did* actively—very actively—have such thoughts.

You also—most actively again—looked for the cake in the market. Bought and paid for it. Brought it home. Unwrapped it. Cut off a piece of it. Ate this piece. Cut off another piece. Ate this one. Refused to put the rest of the cake in the refrigerator. Finished the whole cake. Et-cetera!

So, again, you actively thought about the cake, actively got it and devoured it, and actively felt very good most of the way. Then—later!—you probably lambasted your thoughts, and feelings, and actions, and especially castigated your*self*, or *personhood*, for buying and devouring the damned cake. Whereupon your self-downing helped you to wrongly think and feel that an inadequate person like you could *never* really control your pastry eating habits in the future and therefore you would *always* continue to eat too much cake and other sweet foods.

For the above reasons, and a number of others we could add if we had the space, *Insight No. 3* holds: Because your harmful eating habits usually have a long history, include biological tendencies, are accompanied and impelled by both learned and genetically favored self- defeating thoughts, feelings, and actions, and currently are still actively practiced and practiced, you rarely can find any quick, easy way to change them. No magic. No outside force or influence. No mere seeing and accepting of *Insight No. 1* and of *Insight No. 2*. No, it's not that easy! *Acknowledging* Insights No. 1 and 2 is fine—and is usually a prerequisite to cognitive, emotional and behavioral change. For unless you clearly see that *you* are still largely and actively *keeping* you that way, you probably will never really change. So Insights No. 1 and 2 are very important precursors of change. But insight, as RET has always said, is not enough.

Insight No. 3 straightforwardly insists: Only steady, forceful work and practice—yes, *work and practice!*—will get you to do your self-changing job. Once you keep working, working, working at modifying your irrational, self-defeating thoughts, feelings, and behaviors it may well become easi*er* (though still not just easy) to do so and you may *habitually* tend to think, "I *prefer* to eat ice cream and strawberry shortcake but I never *have* to do so. It's not *awful* but only inconvenient to eat only a small piece today. I *can* stand frustration, though I still won't like it."

And, as you habitually come to create these self-helping thoughts about eating and not eating, you can keep practicing and practicing suitable actions, such as not looking for the ice cream and cake, not buying them, and only having a small portion of them everyday if you do buy them.

As you can see, Insights Nos. 1, 2, and 3 involve strong thinking and rethinking, selective feeling and re-feeling, and action, action, and action. Hard work? Of course. Worth it? Try it and see. Long-range hedonism can decidedly pay off. For a long, long time!

References

Abrams, M. (1991). The eating disorder inventory as a predictor of compliance in a behavioral weight loss program. *International Journal of Eating Disorders, 10,* 355–360.

Adler, A. (1964). *Superiority and social interest.* Evanston, IL: Northwestern University Press.

Allon, N. (1973). The stigma of obesity in everyday life. In Government Printing Office (Ed.). *Obesity in Perspective.* Washington, D.C.

Anderson, J.W., Floore, T.L., Geil, P.B., O'Neal, D.S., & Balm, T.K. (1991). Hypocholesterolemic effects of different bulk–forming hydrophilic fibers as adjuncts to dietary therapy in mild to moderate hypercholesterolemia. *Archives of Internal Medicine, 151,* 1597–1602.

Antonello, J. (1989). *How to become naturally thin by eating more.* New York: Avon Books.

Arjmandi, B.H., Ahn, J., Nathani, S., & Reeves, R.D. (1992). Dietary soluble fiber and cholesterol affect serum cholesterol concentration, hepatic portal venous short-chain fatty acid concentrations and fecal sterol excretion in rats. *Journal of Nutrition, 122,* 246–253.

Atkins, R.C. (1989). *Dr. Atkins' diet revolution.* New York: Bantam Books.

Bandura, A. (1986). *Social foundations of thought and action: A social cognitive theory.* Englewood Cliffs, NJ: Prentice-Hall.

Beck, B., Burlet, A., Nicolas, J., & Burlet, C. (1990). Hypothalamic neuropeptide y (npy) in obese Zucker rats: implications in feeding and sexual behaviors. *Physiology & Behavior, 47,* 449–453.

Bellizzi, J.A., Klassen, M.L., & Belonax, J.J. (1989). Stereotypical beliefs about overweight and smoking and decision-making in assignments to sales territories. *Perceptual & Motor Skills, 69,* 419–429.

Bennett, G.A. (1988). Cognitive-behavioural treatments for obesity. 31st annual conference of the society for psychosomatic research (1987, London, England). *Journal Of Psychosomatic Research, 32,* 661–665.

Bennett, W & Gurin, J. (1991). *The dieter's dilemma.* New York: Basic Books.

Bennett, W. (1987). Dietary treatments of obesity. *Annals of the New York Academy of Sciences, 499,* 250–263.

Bennett, W.I. (1984). Dieting: ideology versus physiology. *Psychiatric Clinics of North America, 7,* 321–334.

Benson, P.L., Severs, D., Tatgenhorst, J., & Loddengaard, N. (1980). The social costs of obesity: a non-reactive field study. *Social Behavior and Personality, 8,* 1, 91–8, 1, 96.

Berger, S.M. (1985). *Dr. Berger's Immune Power Diet.* New York: Signet Books.

*Bernard, M.E. (1986). *Staying alive in an irrational world: Albert Ellis and rational-emotive therapy.* South Melbourne, Australia: Carlson/Macmillan, Secaucus, NJ: Carol Publishing Group.

*Bernard, M.E. (1991). *Using rational-emotive therapy effectively: A practitioner's guide.* New York: Plenum Press.

Bernardis Lee, L., McEwen, G., Kodis, M. & Feldman, M.J. (1987). Pair-feeding of sham-operated controls to rats with dorsomedial hypothalamic lesions: New evidence for an "organismic" set point. *Behavioural Brain Research, 26,* 99–108.

Bernier, M. & Avard, J. (1986). Self-efficacy, outcome, and attrition in a weight-reduction program. *Cognitive Therapy & Research, 10,* 319–338.

Berry, E.M., Hirsch, J., Most, J., & Thornton, J. (1986). The role of dietary fat in human obesity. *International Journal of Obesity, 10,* 123–131.

Bierce, A. (1983). *The collected writings of Ambrose Bierce.* New York: Lyle Stuart.

Blackburn, G.L., Wilson, G.T., Kanders, B.S., Stein, L.J., Lavin, P.T., Adler, J., & Brownell, K.D. (1989). Weight cycling: the experience of human dieters. *American Journal of Clinical Nutrition, 49,* 1105–1109.

Blackburn, G.L. & Kanders, B.S. (1987). Medical evaluation and treatment of the obese patient with cardiovascular disease. *American Journal of Cardiology, 60,* 55G–58G.

Blair, A.J., Lewis, V.J., & Booth, D.A. (1990). Does emotional eating interfere with success in attempts at weight control? *Appetite, 15,* 151–157.

Blundell, J.E. (1990). Appetite disturbance and the problems of overweight. *Drugs, 39 Suppl 3,* 1–19.

Bouchard, C. (1991). Current understanding of the etiology of obesity: genetic and nongenetic factors. *American Journal of Clinical Nutrition, 53,* 1561S–1565S.

*Bourland, D.D.,Jr. & Johnston, P.D. (1991). *To be or not: An E-prime anthology.* San Francisco: International Society for General Semantics.

Bray, G.A. (1987). Overweight is Risking Fate. In R.J. Wurtman & J.J. Wurtman (Eds.). *Human Obesity* (pp. 14–28). New York: Annals of the New York Academy of Sciences.

Briddon, S., Beck, S.A., & Tisdale, M.J. (1991). Changes in activity of lipoprotein lipase, plasma free fatty acids and triglycerides with weight loss in a cachexia model. *Cancer Letter, 57,* 49–53.

Brillat-Savarin, J.A. (1926). *The physiology of taste or meditations on transcendental gastronomy.* New York: Doubleday.

Brown, P.J. & Konner, M. (1987). An anthropological perspective on obesity. *Annals of the New York Academy of Sciences, 499,* 29–46.

Brownell, K.D. (1989). Weight cycling. *American Journal of Clinical Nutrition, 49,* 937.

Brownell, K.D., Greenwood, M.R., Stellar, E., & Shrager, E.E. (1986). The effects of repeated cycles of weight loss and regain in rats. *Physiology and Behavior, 38,* 459–464.

Bruch, H. (1978). *The golden cage.* Cambridge: Harvard University Press.

Bruch, H. (1981). Developmental considerations of anorexia nervosa and obesity. *Canadian Journal of Psychiatry, 26,* 212–217.

Burack, R.C., Keller, J.B., & Higgins, M.W. (1985). Cardiovascular risk factors and obesity: are baseline levels of blood pressure, glucose, cholesterol and uric acid elevated prior to weight gain? *Journal of Chronic Diseases, 38,* 865–872.

*Burns, D.D. (1980). *Feeling good: The new mood therapy.* New York: Morrow.

Cahnman, W.J. (1968). The stigma of obesity. *The Sociological Quarterly, 9:3,* Summer, S299.

Canning, H. & Mayer, J. (1966). Obesity - Its possible effects on college admissions. *New England Journal of Medicine, 275,* 1172–1174.

Cash, T.F. & Hicks, K.L. (1990). Being fat versus thinking fat: relationships with body image, eating behaviors, and well-being. *Cognitive Therapy & Research, 14,* 327–341.

Castro, R.C., Vieira, J.G., Chacra, A.R., Besser, G.M., Grossman, A.B., & Lengyel, A.M. (1990). Pyridostigmine enhances, but does not normalize the GH response to GH-releasing hormone in obese subjects. *Acta Endocrin, 122,* 385–390.

Chambliss, C.A. & Murray, E.J. (1979). Efficacy attribution, locus of control, and weight loss. *Cognitive Therapy & Research, 3,* 349–353.

Chandarana, P.C., Conlon, P., Holliday, R.L., & Deslippe, T. (1990). A prospective study of psychosocial aspects of gastric stapling surgery. *Psychiatric Journal of the University of Ottawa, 15,* 32–35.

Chase, C. (1981). *The great american waistline: Putting it on and keeping it off.* New York: Putnam Group.

Coll, M., Meyer, A., & Stunkard, A.J. (1979). Obesity and food choices in public places. *Archives of General Psychiatry, 36,* 795–797.

Contreras, R.J., King, S., Rives, L., Williams, A., & Wattleton, T. (1991). Dietary obesity and weight cycling in rats: a model of stress-induced hypertension? *American Journal of Physiology, 261,* R848–R857.

Cooper, J.R., Bloom, F.E. & Roth, R.H. (1986). *The biochemical basis of psychopharmacology.* New York: Oxford University Press.

Costanzo, P.R. & Schiffman, S.S. (1989). Thinness—not obesity—has a genetic component. *Neuroscience & Biobehavioral Reviews, 13,* 55–58.

Costanzo, P.R. & Woody, E.Z. (1979). Externality as a function of obesity in children: Pervasive style or eating-specific attribute? *Journal of Personality & Social Psychology, 37,* 2286–2296.

Cové, E. (1923). *My method.* New York: Doubleday, Page.

Crandall, C.S. & Biernat, M. (1990). The ideology of anti-fat attitudes. *Journal of Applied Social Psychology, 20,* 227–243.

Crews, D.E. (1988). Body weight, blood pressure and the risk of total and cardiováscular mortality in an obese population. *Human Biology, 60,* 417–433.

Crisp, A.H. & McGuiness, B. (1976). Jolly fat: Relation between obesity and psychoneurosis in general population. *British Medical Journal, 1,* 7–9.

Daniels, J.S. (1986). The pathogenesis and treatment of obesity. *New Directions For Mental Health Services, 31,* 359.

*Danysh, J. (1974). *Stop without quitting.* San Francisco: International Society for General Semantics.

Davis, J.M., Wheeler, R.W., & Willy, E. (1987). Cognitive correlates of obesity in a nonclinical population. *Psychological Reports, 60,* 1151–1156.

DeJong, W. (1980). The stigma of obesity: the consequences of naive assumptions concerning the causes of physical deviance. *Journal of Health and Social Behavior, 21,* 75–87.

Derksen, J. (1990). An exploratory study of borderline personality disorder in women with eating disorders and psychoactive substance dependent patients. *Journal of Personality Disorders, 4,* 372–380.

*DiGiuseppe, R.(Speaker) (1990). *What do I do with my anger: hold it in or let it out?* New York: Cassette recording. Institute for Rational-Emotive Therapy.

*DiGiuseppe, R.(Speaker) (1991). *Maximizing the moment: How to have more fun and happiness in life.* New York: Cassette Recording. Institute for Rational-Emotive Therapy.

*DiMattia, D.J. et al. (Speakers) (1987). *Mind over myths: Handling difficult situations in the workplace.* New York: Institute for Rational-Emotive Therapy.

*DiMattia, D.J. & Long,S. (Speakers)(1990). *Self-directed sales success.* Cassette recording. New York: Rational Effectiveness Training Systems.

Dritschel, B.H., Williams, K., & Cooper, P.J. (1991). Cognitive distortions amongst women experiencing bulimic episodes. *International Journal of Eating Disorders, 10,* 547–555.

*Dryden, W. (1990). *Dealing with anger problems: Rational-emotive therapeutic interventions.* Sarasota, FL: Professional Resource Exchange.

*Dryden, W. & Hill, H (Eds.) (1992). *The fundamentals of rational-emotive therapy.* Stony Stratford, England: Open University Press.

*Dryden, W. & DiGiuseppe, R. (1990). *A primer on rational-emotive therapy.* Champaign, IL: Research Press.

*Dryden, W. & Gordon, J. (1991). *Think your way to happiness.* London: Sheldon Press.

DuBois, B.C., Goodman, J.D., & Conway, T.L. (1989). Dietary and behavioral prediction of obesity in the navy. *US Naval Health Research Center Report,* Report No 56, p. 35.

DuCoff, J. & Cohen, S.C. (1980). *A guide to health, success and beauty for the woman size 16 or over.* New York: Simon & Schuster.

Dwyer, J. (1980). Sixteen popular diets: Brief nutritional analyses. In A.J. Stunkard (Ed.). *Obesity*, Philadelphia, PA.: W.B. Saunders Company.

Edell, B.H., Edington, S., Herd, B., & O'Brien, R.M. (1987). Self-efficacy and self-motivation predictors of weight loss. Addictive Behaviors, *12*, 63–66.

Elder, G.H. (1969). Appearance and education in marriage mobility. *American Sociological Review, 34*, 519–527.

*Ellis, A. (1962). *Reason and emotion in psychotherapy*. Secaucus, NJ: Citadel.

*Ellis, A. (1972a). *Executive leadership: The rational-emotive approach*. New York: Institute for Rational-Emotive Therapy.

Ellis, A. (1972b). *Psychotherapy and the value of a human being*. New York: Institute for Rational-Emotive Therapy.

*Ellis, A. (1973). *Humanistic psychotherapy: The rational-emotive approach*. New York: McGraw-Hill.

*Ellis, A. (1974). *Technique of disputing irrational beliefs (DIBS)*. New York: Institute for Rational-Emotive Therapy.

*Ellis, A. (1975). *How to live with a neurotic: At home and at work*. CA: Wilshire Brooks. Original edition, 1957.

*Ellis, A. (1976). RET abolishes most of the human ego. *Psychotherapy, 13*, 343–348.

*Ellis, A. (1977). *Anger - How to live with and without it*. Secaucus, NJ: Citadel Press.

Ellis, A. (1985a). Intellectual fascism. *Journal of Rational-Emotive Therapy, 3(1)*, 3–12.

*Ellis, A. (1985b). *Overcoming resistance: Rational-emotive therapy with difficult clients*. New York: Springer.

*Ellis, A. (1988a). *How To stubbornly refuse to make yourself miserable about anything—yes, anything!* Secaucus, NJ: Lyle Stuart.

Ellis, A. (1990). Let's not ignore individuality. *American Psychologist, 45*, 781.

*Ellis, A. (1991a). The revised ABCs of rational-emotive therapy. In J. Zeig (Ed.). *Evolution of psychotherapy* 2nd ed. New York: Brunner/Mazel.

*Ellis, A. (1991b). Using RET effectively: Reflections and interview. In M.E.Bernard (Ed.). *Using rational-emotive therapy effectively* (pp. 1–33). New York: Plenum.

*Ellis, A. (1991c). Achieving self-actualization. In A.Jones & R. Crandall (Ed.). *Handbook of self-actualization.* Corte, Madera, CA: Select Press.

Ellis, A. (1992). Foreword. In P. Hauck (Ed.). *Overcoming the rating game* (pp. 1–4). Louisville, KY: Westminster/John Knox.

*Ellis, A. & Becker, I. (1982). *A guide to personal happiness.* North Hollywood, CA: Wilshire Books.

*Ellis, A. & DiMattia, D. (1991). *Rational effectiveness training: A new method of facilitating management and labor relations.* New York: Institute for Rational-Emotive Therapy.

*Ellis, A. & Dryden, W. (1987). *The practice of rational-emotive therapy.* New York: Springer.

*Ellis, A. & Dryden, W. (1990). *The essential Albert Ellis.* New York: Springer.

*Ellis, A. & Dryden, W. (1991). *A dialogue with Albert Ellis: Against dogma.* Milton Keynes, England: Open University Press.

*Ellis, A. & Harper, R.A. (1975). *A new guide to rational living.* North Hollywood, CA: Wilshire Books.

*Ellis, A. & Harper, R.A.(Speakers) (1990). *A guide to rational living.* Los Angeles: Cassette recording.

*Ellis, A. & Hunter, P. (1991). *Why am I always broke? How to be sane about money.* Secaucus, NJ: Lyle Stuart.

*Ellis, A. & Knaus, W. (1977). *Overcoming procrastination.* New York: New American Library.

*Ellis, A., McInerncy, J.F., DiGiuseppe, R., & Yeager, R.J. (1988). *Rational-emotive therapy with alcoholics and substance abusers.* New York: Pergamon.

*Ellis, A., Vega, G. & DiMattia, D. (1990). *Self-management: Strategies for personal success.* New York: Institute for Rational-Emotive Therapy.

*Ellis, A. & Velten, E. (1992). *When AA doesn't work for you: A rational guide for quitting alcohol.* New York: Barricade Books.

*Ellis, A.(Speaker) (1973a). *How to stubbornly refuse to be ashamed of anything.* New York: Cassette recording. Institute for Rational-Emotive Therapy.

*Ellis, A.(Speaker) (1973b). *Twenty-one ways to stop worrying.* New York: Cassette recording. Institute for Rational Emotive Therapy.

*Ellis, A.(Speaker) (1974). *Rational living in an irrational world.* New York: Cassette recording. Institute for Rational-Emotive Therapy.

*Ellis, A.(Speaker) (1975). *RET and assertiveness training.* New York: Cassette recording. Institute for Rational-Emotive Therapy.

*Ellis, A.(Speaker) (1976). *Conquering low frustration tolerance.* New York: Cassette recording. Institute for Rational-Emotive Therapy.

*Ellis, A.(Speaker) (1977a). *Conquering the dire need for love.* New York: Cassette recording. Institute for Rational-Emotive Therapy.

*Ellis, A.(Speaker) (1977b). *A garland of rational humorous songs.* New York: Cassette recording. Institute for Rational-Emotive Therapy.

*Ellis, A.(Speaker) (1978). *I'd like to stop but . . . Dealing with addictions.* New York: Cassette recording. Institute for Rational-Emotive Therapy.

*Ellis, A.(Speaker) (1980). *Twenty-two ways to brighten up your love life.* New York: Cassette recording. Institute for Rational-Emotive Therapy.

*Ellis, A.(Speaker) (1988). *Unconditionally accepting yourself and others.* New York: Cassette recording. Institute for Rational-Emotive Therapy.

*Ellis, A.(Speaker) (1990b). *Albert Ellis live at the Learning Annex.* New York: 2 cassettes. Institute for Rational-Emotive Therapy.

*Ellis, A.(Speaker) (1991). *How to refuse to be angry, vindictive, and unforgiving.* New York: Cassette recording. Institute for Rational-Emotive Therapy.

English, C. (1991). Food is my best friend: self-justifications and weight loss efforts. *Research in the Sociology of Health Care,* 9, 335–9, 345.

Ernsberger, P. & Haskew, P. (1986). Correspondence: News about obesity. *The New England Journal of Medicine, 315,* 130–131.

Ernsberger, P. & Haskew, P. (1987). Health implications of obesity: An alternate view. *Journal of Obesity and Weight Regulation,* 6, 58–137.

Facchinetti, F., Giovannini, C., Barletta, C., & Petraglia, F. (1986). Hyperendorphinemia in obesity and relationships to affective state. *Physiology & Behavior, 36,* 937–940.

Fantino M., Faion, F., & Rolland, Y. (1986). Effect of dex-fenfluramine on body weight set-point: Study in the rat with hoarding behaviour. *Appetite, 251,* 91–96.

Faust, I.M., Johnson, P.R., & Hirsch, J. (1980). Long-term effects of early nutritional experience on the development of obesity in the rat. *Journal of Nutrition, 110,* 2027–2034.

Faust, I.M., Johnson, P.R., Stern, J.S., & Hirsch, J. (1978). Diet-induced adipocyte number increase in adult rats: a new model of obesity. *American Journal of Physiology, 235,* E279–E286.

Fitzgibbon, M.L. & Kirschenbaum, D.S. (1990). Heterogeneity of clinical presentation among obese individuals seeking treatment. *Addictive Behaviors, 15,* 291–295.

Foster, G.D., Wadden, T.A., Feurer, I.D., Jennings, A.S., Stunkard, A.J., Crosby, L.O., Ship, J., & Mullen, J.L. (1990). Controlled trial of the metabolic effects of a very-low-calorie diet: short- and long-term effects. *American Journal of Clinical Nutrition, 51,* 167–172.

Frisch, R.E. (1988). Fatness and fertility. *Scientific American, 258,* 88–95.

Fuller, R.W. & Yen, T.T. (1987). The place of animal models and animal experimentation in the study of food intake regulation and obesity in humans. *Annals of the New York Academy of Sciences, 499,* 167–178.

Ganley, R.M. (1989). Emotion and eating in obesity: a review of the literature. *International Journal of Eating Disorders, 8,* 343–361.

Gardier, A.M., Jrouvin, I.H., Orosco, M., Nicolaidis, S., & Jacquot, J. (1989). Effects of food intake and body weight on a serotonergic turnover index in rat hypothalamus. *Brain Research Bulletin, 22,* 531–535.

Garner, D.M., Garfinkel, P.E. & Moldofsky, H. (1978). Perceptual experiences in anorexia nervosa and obesity. *Canadian Psychiatric Association Journal, 23,* 249–263.

*Garner, D. & Wooley, S. (1991). Confronting the failure of behavioral and dietary treatments for obesity. *Clinical Psychology Review, 11,* 729–780.

Garner, D.M. & Olmstead, M.P. (1984). *The Eating Disorders Inventory Manual.* Los Angeles: Western Psychological Services.

Giannini, A., DiRusso, L., Folts, D.J., & Cerimele, G. (1990). Nonverbal communication in moderately obese females: A pilot study. *Annals of Clinical Psychiatry, 2,* 111–113.

Giovannini, C., Ciucci, E., Cassetta, M.R., Cugini, P., & Facchinetti, F. (1991). Unresponsiveness of the endorphinergic system to its physiological feedback in obesity. *Appetite, 16,* 3943.

Giugliano, D., Cozzolino, D., Torella, R., Lefebvre, P.J., Franchimont, P., & D'Onofrio, F. (1991). Persistence of altered metabolic responses to beta-endorphin after normalization of body weight in human obesity. *Acta Endocrinologica, 124,* 159–165.

Goldblatt, P.B., Moore, M.E., & Stunkard, A.J. (1992). Obesity, social class, and mental illness. *Journal of the American Medical Association, 192,* 1039–1044.

Goodman, N.S., Donbusch, S.M., Richardson, S.A., & Hastorf, A.H. (1963). Variant reactions to physical disabilities. *American Sociological Review, 28,* 429–435.

Graham, B., Chang, S., Lin, D., Yakubu, F., & Hill, J.O. (1990). Effect of weight cycling on susceptibility to dietary obesity. *American Journal of Physiology, 259,* R1096–R1102.

Greenberg, B.R. & Harvey, P.D. (1987). Affective lability versus depression as determinants of binge eating. *Addictive Behaviors, 12*, 357–361.

Grossman, S.P. (1984). Contemporary problems concerning our understanding of brain mechanisms that regulate food intake and body weight. In A.J. Stunkard & E. Stellar (Eds.). *Eating and its disorders* (pp. 5–14). New York: Raven Press.

Groves, P.M. & Rebec, G.V. (1988). *Introduction to biological psychology*. Dubuque, Iowa: Wm. C. Brown.

Hallonquist, J.D. & Brandes, J.S. (1984). Ventromedial hypothalamic lesions in rats: Gradual elevation of body weight setpoint. *Physiology & Behavior, 33*, 831–836.

Hallstrom, T. & Noppa, H. (1981). Obesity in women in relation to mental illness, social factors and personality traits. *Journal of Psychosomatic Research, 25*, 75–82.

Hankins, N.E. & Hopkins, L. (1978). Locus of control and weight loss in joiners and non-joiners of weight reduction organizations. *Psychological Reports, 43*, 11–14.

Harris Ruth, B. & Martin Roy, J. (1984). Lipostatic theory of energy balance: Concepts and signals. *Nutrition & Behavior, 1*, 253–275.

Harris, M.B. (1990). Is love seen as different for the obese? *Journal of Applied Social Psychology, 20*, 1209–1224.

Harris, M.B. & Smith, S. (1982). Beliefs about obesity: effects of age, ethnicity, sex and weight. *Psychological Reports, 51*, 1055.

Harris, R.B. & Martin, R.J. (1989). Changes in lipogenesis and lipolysis associated with recovery from reversible obesity in mature female rats. *Proceedings of the Society of Experimental Biology & Medicine, 191*, 82–89.

*Hauck, P.A. (1973). *Overcoming depression*. Philadelphia: Westminster.

*Hauck, P.A. (1974). *Overcoming frustration and anger*. Philadelphia: Westminster.

*Hauck, P.A. (1992). *Overcoming the rating game: Beyond self-love - beyond self-esteem*. Louisville, KY: Westminster/John Knox.

Hayakawa, S.I. (1962). *General semantics: The use and misuse of language*. Greenwich, Conn.: Fawcett.

Hays, S.E., Goodwin, F.K., & Paul, S.M. (1981). Cholecystokinin receptors in brain: Effects of obesity, drug treatment, and lesions. *Peptides, 2 Suppl 1*, 21–26.

Heller, R.F. (1991). *The carbohydrate addict's diet*. New York: Dutton Books.

Hendry, L.B. & Gillies, P. (1978). Body type, body esteem, school, and leisure: a study of overweight, average, and underweight adolescents. *Journal of Youth and Adolescence*, June 7, 2, J195.

Herman, C., (1978). Distractibility in dieters and nondieters: An alternative view of "externality". *Journal of Personality & Social Psychology, 36*, 536–548.

Herman, C. & Mack, D. (1975). Restrained and unrestrained eating. *Journal of Personality, 43*, 647–660.

Herman, C., Olmsted, M.P., & Polivy, J. (1983). Obesity, externality, and susceptibility to social influence: An integrated analysis. *Journal of Personality & Social Psychology, 45*, 926–934.

Herman, C.P. & Polivy, J. (1984). A boundary model for the regulation of eating. In A.J. Stunkard & E. Stellar (Eds.). *Eating and its disorders* (pp. 141–156). New York: Raven Press.

Hiller, D.V. (1981). The salience of overweight in personality characterization. *The Journal of Psychology, 2*, 240.

Hiller, D.V. (1982). Overweight as master status: a replication. *The Journal of Psychology, 1*, 113.

Hoebel, B.G. (1984). Neurotransmitters in the control of feeding and its rewards: Monoamines, opiates band brain-gut peptides. In A.J. Stunkard & E. Stellar (Eds.). *Eating and its disorders* (pp. 15–38). New York: Raven Press.

Holub, K. (1987). Sculpting down to size. *The Toronto Star, Dec 7*, C1–C2.

Howard, B.V., Bogardus, C., Ravussin, E., Foley, J.E., Lillioja, S., Mott, D.M., Bennett, P.H., & Knowler, W.C. (1991). Studies of the etiology of obesity in Pima Indians. *American Journal of Clinical Nutrition, 53*, 1577S–1585S.

Industry Week (1974). Fat Execs get slimmer paychecks. *180*, 21–24.

Institute for Scientific Information (1991). To attack obesity, Rockefeller University's Jules Hirsch calls for a blend of new biology and clinical medicine. *Science Watch, 2*, 3–7.

Jacobson, E. (1938). *You must relax.* New York: McGraw-Hill.

Jasper, C.R. & Klassen, M.L. (1990a). Perceptions of salespersons' appearance and evaluation of job performance. *Perceptual & Motor Skills, 71*, 563–566.

Jasper, C.R. & Klassen, M.L. (1990b). Stereotypical beliefs about appearance: implications for retailing and consumer issues. *Perceptual & Motor Skills, 71*, 519–528.

Jebb, S.A., Goldberg, G.R., Coward, W.A., Murgatroyd, P.R., & Prentice, A.M. (1991). Effects of weight cycling caused by intermittent dieting on metabolic rate and body composition in obese women. *International Journal of Obesity, 15*, 367–374.

Jeffery, R.W. & Wing, R.R. (1983). Recidivism and self-cure of smoking and obesity: data from population studies. *American Psychologist, 38*, 852.

Jenkins, D.J., Ocana, A., Jenkins, A.L., Wolever, T.M., Vuksan, V., Katzman, L., Hollands, M., Greenberg, G., Corey, P., & Patten, R. (1992). Metabolic advantages of spreading the nutrient load: effects of increased meal frequency in non-insulin-dependent diabetes. *American Journal of Clinical Nutrition, 55*, 461–467.

Johnson, E.H. (1990). Interrelationships between psychological factors, overweight, and blood pressure in adolescents. *Journal of Adolescent Health Care, 11*, 310–318.

Johnson, S.F., Swenson, W.M., & Gastineau, C.F. (1976). personality characteristics in obesity: relation of MMPI profile and age of onset of obesity to success in weight reduction. *American Journal of Clinical Nutrition*, Jun-J32.

Johnson, W. (1946). *People in quandaries.* New York: Harper & Row.

Kallen, D.J. & Doughty, A. (1984). The relationship of weight, the self perception of weight and self esteem with courtship behavior. *Marriage and Family Review, 7*, 1–2, Spring.

Kasset, J.A., Gershon, E.S., Maxwell, M., & Goroff, J.J. (1988). Psychiatric disorders in the first-degree relatives of probands with bulimia nervosa. *American Journal of Psychiatry, 146,* 1468–1471.

Kathan, M. (1989). *The T-Factor Diet.* New York: W.W. Norton & Company.

Keefe, P.H., Wyshograd, D., & Weinberger, E. (1984). Binge eating and outcome of behavioral treatment of obesity: A preliminary report. *Behavior Research and Therapy, 22,* 319–324.

Keesey, R.E. (1988). The body-weight set point. What can you tell your patients? *Post Graduate Medicine, 83,* 114–118.

Keesey, R.E. (1989). Physiological regulation of body weight and the issue of obesity. *Medical Clinics North America, 73,* 15–27.

Keesey, R.E. & Corbett, S.W. (1985). Metabolic defense of the body weight setpoint. In A.J. Stunkard & E. Stellar (Eds.). *Eating and its disorders* (pp. 87–96). New York: Raven Press.

Keller, U. (1990). Drugs against obesity. *TherUmsch, 47,* 658–663.

Kendler, K.S., MacLean, C., Neale, M., Kessler, R., Heath, A., & Eaves, L. (1991). The genetic epidemiology of bulimia nervosa. *American Journal of Psychiatry, 148,* 1627–1637.

Keys, A. (1989). Longevity of man: relative weight and fatness in middle age. *Annals of Medicine, 21,* 163–168.

Keys, A. (1986). Is there an ideal body weight. *British Medical Journal, 293,* 1023–1024.

Keys, A., Menotti, A., Karvonen, M.J., Aravanis, C., Blackburn, H., Buzina, R., Djordjevic, B.S., Dontas, A.S., Fidanza, F., & Keys, M.H. (1986). The diet and 15-year death rate in the seven countries study. *American Journal of Epidemiology, 124,* 903–915.

Keys, A., Brozek, J., Henschel, A., Mickelson, O. & Taylor, H.C. (1950). *The biology of human starvation.* Minneapolis: University of Minnesota Press.

Kincey, J. (1983). Compliance with a behavioural weight-loss programme: target setting and locus of control. *Behaviour Research & Therapy, 21,* 109–114.

Kittel, F., Rustin, R.M., Dramaix, M., DeBacker, G., & Kornitzer, M. (1978). Psycho-socio-biological correlates of moderate overweight in an industrial population. *Journal of Psychosomatic Research, 22*, 145–158.

Kleinke, C. & Staneski, R. (1980). First impressions of female bust size. *Journal of Social Psychology, 110*, 123–134.

Klesges, R.C. (1983). An analysis of body image distortions in a nonpatient population. *International Journal of Eating Disorders, 2*, 35–41.

Klesges, R.C., Eck, L.H., Hanson, C.L., & Haddock, C. (1990). Effects of obesity, social interactions, and physical environment on physical activity in preschoolers. *Health Psychology, 9*, 435–449.

Klyde, B.J. & Hirsch, J. (1979). Increased cellular proliferation in adipose tissue of adult rats fed a high-fat diet. *Journal of Lipid Research, 20*, 705–715.

*Knaus, W.(Speaker) (1975). *Overcoming procrastination.* New York: Cassette recording. Institute for Rational-Emotive Therapy.

Kohn, I.J. & Ribeiro, L.G. (1991). The role of cholesterol in atherosclerosis and its potential management by dietary fiber. *Arq Bras Cardiol, 56*, 173–184.

*Korzybski, A. (1933). *Science and sanity.* San Francisco: International Society of General Semantics.

Kozlowski, L.T. & Schachter, S. (1975). Effects of cue prominence and palatability on the drinking behavior of obese and normal humans. *Journal of Personality & Social Psychology, 32*, 1055–1059.

Kraemer, H.C., Berkowitz, R.I., & Hammer, L.D. (1990a). Methodological difficulties in studies in obesity: i. measurement issues. *Annals of Behavioral Medicine, 12*, 112–118.

Kraemer, H.C., Berkowitz, R.I., & Hammer, L.D. (1990b). Methodological difficulties in studies of obesity: ii. design and analysis issues. *Annals of Behavioral Medicine, 12*, 119–124.

Kraft, K. & Vetter, H. (1991). Long-term opiate receptor antagonism in a patient with panhypopituitarism: effects on appetite, prolactin and demand for vasopressin. *Hormonal and Metabolic Research*, *23*, 74–75.

Krieshok, S.I. & Karpowitz, D.H. (1988). A review of selected literature on obesity and guidelines for treatment. *Journal of Counseling & Development*, *66*, 326–330.

Lapidus, L., Bengtsson, C., Hallstrom, T., & Bjorntorp, P. (1989). Obesity adipose tissue distribution and health in women—results from a population study in Gothenburg, Sweden. *Appetite*, *13*, 25–35.

LaPorte, D.J. (1990). A fatiguing effect in obese patients during partial fasting: Increase in vulnerability to emotion-related events and anxiety. *International Journal of Eating Disorders*, *9*, 345–355.

Larkin, J. & Pines, H.A. (1979). No fat persons need apply: Experimental studies of the overweight stereotype and hiring preference. *Sociology of Work and Occupations*, *6*, 312–327.

Larsen, F. (1990). Psychosocial function before and after gastric banding surgery for morbid obesity: a prospective psychiatric study. *Acta Psychiatrica Scandinavica*, *82*, 57.

Larsen, F. & Torgersen, S. (1989). Personality changes after gastric banding surgery for morbid obesity. A prospective study. *Journal of Psychosomatic Research*, *33*, 323–334.

*Lazarus, R.S. & Folkman, S. (1984). *Stress, appraisal, and coping*. New York: Springer.

Leander, J.D. (1987). Fluoxetine suppresses palatability-induced ingestion. *Psychopharmacology*, *91*, 285–287.

Leibel, R.L., Berry, E.M., & Hirsch, J. (1991). Metabolic and hemodynamic responses to endogenous and exogenous catecholamines in formerly obese subjects. *American Journal of Physiology*, *260*, R785–R791.

Leibel, R.L. & Hirsch, J. (1984). Diminished energy requirements in reduced-obese patients. *Metabolism*, *33*, 164–170.

Leibel, R.L. & Hirsch, J. (1985). Metabolic characterization of obesity. *Annals of Internal Medicine*, *103*, 1000–1002.

Leibel, R.L. & Hirsch, J. (1987). Site- and sex-related differences in adrenoreceptor status of human adipose tissue. *Journal of Clinical Endocrinology and Metabolism*, *64*, 1205–1210.

Leon, G., Eckert, E.D., Teed, D., & Buchwald, H. (1979). Changes in body image and other psychological factors after intestinal bypass surgery for massive obesity. *Journal of Behavioral Medicine*, Mar, 2–1, 55.

Lerner, M.J. (1980). *The belief in a just world*. New York: Plenum Press.

Levine, L.R., Enas, G.G., Thompson, W.L., Byyny, R.L., Dauer, A.D., Kirby, R.W., Kreindler, T.G., Levy, B., Lucas, C.P., & McIlwain, H.H. (1989). Use of fluoxetine, a selective serotonin-uptake inhibitor, in the treatment of obesity: a dose-response study (with a commentary by Michael Weintraub). *International Journal of Obesity*, 13, 635–645.

Lowe, M.R. & Fisher, E.B. (1983). Emotional reactivity, emotional eating, and obesity: a naturalistic study. *Journal of Behavioral Medicine*, 6, 135–149.

Lowe, M.R. & Fisher, E. B. (1988). Restraint, disinhibition, hunger and negative affect eating. *Addictive Behaviors*, 13, 369–377.

Lynn, M. & Shurgot, B. (1984). Responses to lonely hearts advertisements: Effects of reported physical attractiveness, physique, and coloration. *Personality and Social Psychology Bulletin*, 10, 349–357.

Maddox, G.L., Back, K., & Liederman, V. (1968). Overweight as social deviance and disability. *Journal of Health and Social Behavior*, 9, 287–298.

Marcus, M.D., Wing, R.R., Ewing, L. & Kern, E. (1990). A double-blind, placebo-controlled trial of fluoxetine plus behavior modification in the treatment of obese binge-eaters and non-binge-eaters. *American Journal of Psychiatry*, 147, 876–881.

Marcus, M.D., Wing, R.R., & Hopkins, J. (1988). Obese binge eaters: affect, cognitions, and response to behavioral weight control. *Journal of Consulting & Clinical Psychology*, 56, 433–439.

Marlatt, G.A. & Gordon, J.R. (1985). *Relapse prevention*. New York: Guilford Press.

Marshall, J.R. & Neill, J. (1977). The removal of a psychosomatic symptom: Effects on the marriage. *Family Process*, Sep, *16–3*, 280.

Mathus Vliegen, E.M.H., Tytgat, G.N.J., & Veldhuyzen Offermans, E.A.M.L. (1990). Intragastric balloon in the treatment of super-morbid obesity. Double-blind, sham-controlled, crossover evaluation of 500-milliliter balloon. *Gastroenterology*, 99, 362–369.

Mayer, J. (1953). Genetic, traumatic and environmental factors in the etiology of obesity. *Physiological Review*, 33, 472–508.

Mayer, J. (1968). *Overweight: Causes, cost, and control.* Englewood Cliffs, N.J.

Maykovich, M.K. (1978). Social constraints in eating patterns among the obese and overweight. *Social Problems*, 25, 453–460.

Mazel, J. (1982). *The Beverly Hills diet.* New York: Berkley Books.

McClelland, L., Mynors, W., Fahy, T., & Treasure, J. (1991). Sexual abuse, disordered personality and eating disorders. *British Journal of Psychiatry*, 158, 63–68.

Meichenbaum, D. (1977). *Cognitive-behavior modification.* New York: Plenum.

Melby, C.L., Schmidt, W.D., & Corrigan, D. (1990). Resting metabolic rate in weight-cycling collegiate wrestlers compared with physically active, noncycling control subjects. *American Journal of Clinical Nutrition*, 52, 409–414.

Meyer, A.W., Stunkard, A.J. & Coll, M. (1980). Food accessibility and food choice. A test of Schacter's externality hypothesis. *Archives of General Psychiatry*, 37, 1133–1135.

Miller, C.T., Rothblum, E.D., Barbour, L., & Brand, P.A. (1990). Social interactions of obese and nonobese women. *Journal of Personality*, 58, 365–380.

Miller, K.J. (1991). Childhood sexual abuse as a factor in eating disorders in women: prevalence and symptom severity. *Dissertation Abstracts International*, 51, 5582–5583.

Miller, P.M. (1983). *The Hilton Head metabolism diet.* New York: Warner Books.

Mills, J.K. (1991). Differences in locus of control between obese adult and adolescent females undergoing weight reduction. *Journal of Psychology, 125*, 195–197.

Mitchell, J.E. & Pyle, R.L. (1988). The diagnosis and clinical characteristics of bulimia. In B.J. Blinder, B.F. Chaitlin & R.S. Goldstein (Eds.). *The Eating Disorders* (pp. 267–273). New York: PMA Publishing Corp.

Moore, R., Mills, I.H., & Forster, A. (1981). Naloxone in the treatment of anorexia nervosa: Effect on weight gain and lipolysis. *Journal of the Royal Society of Medicine, 74*, 129–131.

Morley, J.E. (1989). An approach to the development of drugs for appetite disorders. *Neuropsychobiology, 21*, 22–30.

Nachman, M. (1959). The inheritance of saccharin preference. *Journal of Comparative & Physiological Psychology, 52*, 451–457.

Nasser, M. (1988). Culture and weight consciousness. *Journal of Psychosomatic Research, 32*, 573–577.

Neggers, Y.H., Stitt, K.R., & Roseman, J.M. (1990). Obesity: problems with definition and prevalence. *Journal of Obesity & Weight Regulation, 8*, 119–135.

Ness, R., Laskarzewski, P., & Price, R.A. (1991). Inheritance of extreme overweight in black families. *Human Biology, 63*, 39–52.

Nir, Z. & Neumann, L. (1991). Self-esteem, internal-external locus of control, and their relationship to weight reduction. *Journal of Clinical Psychology, 47*, 568–575.

Nisbett, R.E. (1972). Hunger, obesity, and the ventromedial hypothalamus. *Psychological Review, 79(6)*, 433–453.

Ogles, B.M., Lambert, M.J., & Craig, D.E. (1991). Comparison of self-help books for coping with loss: Expectations and attributions. *Journal of Consulting Psychology, 38*, 387–393.

Ono, K., Kawamura, K., Shimizu, N. & Ito, C. (1990). Fetal hypothalamic brain grafts to the ventromedial hypothalamic obese rats: an immunohistochemical, electrophysiological and behavioral study. *Brain Research Bulletin, 24*, 89–96.

Pargaman, D. (1969). The incidence of obesity among college students. *Journal of School Health, 29*, 621–625.

Pasquali, R., Besteghi, L., Casimirri, F., & Melchionda, N. (1990). Mechanisms of action of the intragastric balloon in obesity: Effects on hunger and satiety. *Appetite, 15,* 3–11.

Peck, A.M. & Vagero, D.H. (1989). Adult body height, self-perceived health and mortality in the Swedish population. *Journal of Epidemiology and Community Health, 43,* 380–384.

Pettitt, D.J., Bennett, P.H., Saad, M.F., Charles, M.A., Nelson, R.G., & Knowler, W.C. (1991). Abnormal glucose tolerance during pregnancy in Pima Indian women. Long-term effects on offspring. *Diabetes, 40 Suppl 2,* 126–130.

Polivy, J. & Herman, C. (1976). Clinical depression and weight change: A complex relation. *Journal of Abnormal Psychology, 85,* 338–340.

Polivy, J., Herman, C., & Warsh, S. (1978a). Internal and external components of emotionality in restrained and unrestrained eaters. *Journal of Abnormal Psychology, 87,* 497–504.

Polivy, J. & Herman, P.C. (1983). *Breaking the diet habit.* New York: Basic Books, Inc.

Pollack Seid, R. (1989). *Never too thin: Why women are at war with their bodies.* New York: Prentice Hall Press.

Presta, E., Leibel, R.L., & Hirsch, J. (1990). Regional changes in adrenergic receptor status during hypocaloric intake do not predict changes in adipocyte size or body shape. *Metabolism, 39,* 307–315.

Price, R.A., Cadoret, R.J., Stunkard, A.J., & Troughton, E. (1987). Genetic contributions to human fatness: An adoption study. *American Journal of Psychiatry, 144,* 1003–1008.

Rabkin, S.W. (1982). Psychosocial determinants of weight reduction in overweight individuals. *Journal of Obesity & Weight Regulation, 2,* 97–106.

Rand, C.S. & Kuldau, J.M. (1990). The epidemiology of obesity and self-defined weight problem in the general population: gender, race, age, and social class. *International Journal of Eating Disorders, 9,* 329–343.

Ravussin, E. & Bogardus, C. (1990). Energy expenditure in the obese: Is there a thrifty gene? *Infusionstherapie, 17,* 108–112.

Reed, D.R., Contreras, R.J., Maggio, C., Greenwood, M.R., & Rodin, J. (1988). Weight cycling in female rats increases dietary fat selection and adiposity. *Physiology and Behavior, 42,* 389–395.

Riccardi, G. & Rivellese, A.A. (1991). Effects of dietary fiber and carbohydrate on glucose and lipoprotein metabolism in diabetic patients. *Diabetes Care, 14,* 1115–1125.

Richardson, S.A., Goodman, N., Hastorf, A.H., & Dornbusch, S.M. (1963). Cultural uniformity in reaction to physical disabilities. *American Sociological Review, 28,* 429–435.

Robert, J.J., Orosco, M., Rouch, C. & Jacquot, C. (1989). Effects of opiate agonists and an antagonist on food intake and brain neurotransmitters in normophagic and obese "cafeteria" rats. *Pharmacology, Biochemistry & Behavior, 34,* 577–583.

Rodin, J. (1981). Current status of the internal-external hypothesis for obesity: what went wrong? *American Psychologist, 36,* 361–372.

Rodin, J., Radke Sharpe, N., Rebuffe Scrive, M., & Greenwood, M.R. (1990). Weight cycling and fat distribution. *International Journal of Obesity, 14,* 303–310.

Rodin, J. & Slochower, J. (1976). Externality in the nonobese: Effects of environmental responsiveness on weight. *Journal of Personality & Social Psychology, 33,* 338–344.

Roe, D.A. & Eickwort, K.R. (1976). Relationships between obesity and associated health factors with unemployment among low income women. *Journal of the American Medical Women's Association, 31,* 193–204.

Ross, C.E. & Mirowsky, J. (1983). Social epidemiology of overweight: A substantive and methodological investigation. *Journal of Health and Social Behavior,* Sep 24–3, 298.

Rothblum, E.D., Brand, P.A., Miller, C.T., & Oetjen, H.A. (1990). The relationship between obesity, employment discrimination, and employment-related victimization. *Journal of Vocational Behavior, 37,* 251–266.

Rozin, P. & Fallon, A. (1988). Body image, attitudes towards weight, and misperceptions of figure preferences of the opposite sex: A comparison of men and women in two generations. *Journal of Abnormal Psychology*, 97, 342–345.

Saad, M.F., Knowler, W.C., Pettitt, D.J., Nelson, R.G., Mott, D.M., & Bennett, P.H. (1990). Insulin and hypertension. Relationship to obesity and glucose intolerance in Pima Indians. *Diabetes*, 39, 1430–1435.

Saland, L.C., Wallace, J.A., Reyes, E., Samora, A., Maez, D., & Comunas, F. (1987). Effects of the serotonin-uptake inhibitor, fluoxetine on immunoreactive serotonin innervation in the rat pituitary gland. *Brain Research Bulletin*, 19, 261–267.

Sampson, E.E. (1989). The challenge of social change in psychology. Globalization and psychology's theory of the person. *American Psychologist*, 44, 914–921.

Sanacora, G., Kershaw, M., Finkelstein, J.A., & White, J.D. (1990). Increased hypothalamic content of preproneuropeptide Y messenger ribonucleic acid in genetically obese Zucker rats and its regulation by food deprivation. *Endocrinology*, 127, 730–737.

Scavo, D., Barletta, C., Vagiri, D., Burla, F., Fontana, M., & Lazzari, R. (1990). Hyperendorphinemia in obesity is not related to the affective state. *Physiology and Behavior*, 48, 681–683.

Schacter, S. & Rodin, J. (1974). *Obese humans and rats*. Washington, D.C.: Erlbaum/Halstead.

Schmidt, U. (1989). Behavioural psychotherapy of eating disorders. special issue: behavioural psychotherapy into the 1990's. *International Review of Psychiatry*, 1, 245–256.

Schneider, B.S., Monahan, J.W., & Hirsch, J. (1979). Brain cholecystokinin and nutritional status in rats and mice. *Journal of Clinical Investigation*, 64, 1348–1356.

Schotte, D.E., Cools, J., & McNally, R.J. (1990). Film-induced negative affect triggers overeating in restrained eaters. *Journal of Abnormal Psychology*, 99, 317–320.

Schotte, D.E. & Stunkard, A.J. (1987). Bulimia vs bulimic behaviors on a college campus. *Journal of the American Medical Association, 258,* 1213–1215.

Schwartz, H. (1986). *Never satisfied.* New York: The Free Press.

Sclafani, A. (1984). Animal models of obesity: Classification and characterization. *International Journal of Obesity, 8,* 491–508.

Sclafani, A. (1987). Dietary-induced overeating. *Annals of the New York Academy of Sciences, 575,* 281–9.

Sclafani, A. & Kluge, L. (1974). Food motivation and body weight levels in hypothalamic hyperphage rats: a dual lipostat model of hunger and appetite. *Journal of Comparative and Physiological Psychology, 86,* 28–46.

Sclafani, A. & Springer, D. (1976). Dietary obesity in adult rats: similarities to hypothalamic and human obesity syndromes. *Physiology and Behavior, 17,* 461–471.

Scogin, F., Jamison, C., & Gochneur, K. (1989). Comparative efficacy of cognitive and behavioral bibliotherapy. *Journal of Consulting and Clinical Psychology, 57,* 403–407.

Seligman, J., Joseph, N., Donovan, J., & Gosnell, M. (1987). The little dieters. *Newsweek, July 27,* 48.

Shelton, H.M. (1991). *Fasting can save your life.* Tampa, Fl.: American Natural Hygiene Society.

Sheppard, K. (1989). *Food addiction: The body knows.* Deerfield Beach, FL.: Health Communications Inc.

*Sichel, J. & Ellis, A. (1984). *RET self-help form.* New York: Institute for Rational-Emotive Therapy.

Silverstein, B., Peterson, B., & Perdue, L. (1986). Some correlates of the thin standard and bodily attractiveness in women. *International Journal of Eating Disorders, 5,* 145–159.

Sims, E.A. & Horton, E.S. (1968). Endocrine and metabolic adaptation to obesity and starvation. *American Journal of Clinical Nutrition,* Dec-D70.

Skouge, J.W. (1990). The biochemistry and development of adipose tissue and the pathophysiology of obesity as it relates to liposuction surgery. *Dermatology Clinics, 8,* 385–393.

Slochower, J. (1976). Emotional labeling and overeating in obese and normal weight individuals. *Psychosomatic Medicine, 38,* 131–139.

Smart, M.S. & Smart, R.C. (1971). On Schachter on obesity. *American Psychologist, 26,* 935–936.

Smith, J.E., Waldor, V.A., & Trembath, D.L. (1990). "Single white male looking for thin, very attractive . . ." *Sex Roles, 23,* 675–685.

Sobal, J. (1984a). Marriage, obesity and dieting. *Marriage and Family Review, 7,* 115–139.

Sobal, J. (1984b). Group dieting, the stigma of obesity, and overweight adolescents: contributions of Natalie Allon to the sociology of obesity. *Marriage and Family Review, 7,* 9–20.

Sobal, J. & Stunkard, A.J. (1989). Socioeconomic status and obesity: A review of the literature. *Psychological Bulletin, 105,* 260–275.

Sommer, B. (1987). *Not another diet book: A right brain program for successful weight management.* Claremont, CA.: Hunter House.

Sonne, H., Sorensen, T.I., Jensen, G., & Schnohr, P. (1989). Influence of fatness, intelligence, education and sociodemographic factors on response rate in a health survey. *Journal of Epidemiology & Community Health, 43,* 369–374.

Sorensen, T.I.A., Sonne, H., Christensen, U., & Kreiner, M. (1982). Reduced intellectual performance in extreme overweight. *Human Biology, 54,* 765–775.

Sorensen, T.I.A. & Sonne, H.S. (1985). Intelligence test performance in obesity in relation to educational attainment and parental social class. *Journal of Biosocial Science, 17,* 379–387.

Stake, J. & Lauer, M. (1987). The consequences of being overweight: A controlled study of gender differences. *Sex Roles, 17,* 31–47.

Stanley, B.G., Kyrkouli, S.E., Lampert, S., & Leibowitz, S.F. (1986). Neuropeptide Y chronically injected into the hypothalamus: a powerful neurochemical inducer of hyperphagia and obesity. *Peptides, 7,* 1189–1192.

Starker, S. (1988). Do-it-yourself therapy. *Psychotherapy*, 25, 142–146.

Steen, S.N., Oppliger, R.A., & Brownell, K.D. (1988). Metabolic effects of repeated weight loss and regain in adolescent wrestlers. *Journal of the American Medical Association, 260*, 47–50.

Steiger, H., Liquornik, K., Chapman, J., & Hussain, N. (1991). Personality and family disturbances in eating-disorder patients: comparison of "restricters" and "bingers" to normal controls. *International Journal of Eating Disorders, 10*, 501–512.

Stillman, I. (1967). *The doctor's quick weight loss diet*. New York: Prentice Hall.

Stricker, E.M. & Verbalis, J.G. (1987). Biological bases of hunger and satiety. *Annals of Behavioral Medicine, 9*, 3–8.

Stunkard, A.J. (1976) *The pain of obesity*, Palo Alto: Bull Publishing.

Stunkard, A.J. (1982). Anorectic agents lower a body weight set point. *Life Science, 30*, 2043–2055.

Stunkard, A.J. (1983). Nutrition, aging and obesity: a critical review of a complex relationship. *International Journal of Obesity, 7*, 201–220.

Stunkard, A.J. (1984). The current status of treatment for obesity in adults. *Res Publ Assoc Res Nerv Ment Dis, 62*, 157–173.

Stunkard, A.J. (1985). Behavioural management of obesity, *Medical Journal of Australia, 142*, S13–S20.

Stunkard, A.J. (1988). The Salmon lecture. Some perspectives on human obesity: its causes. *Bulletin of NY Academy of Medicine, 64*, 902–923.

Stunkard, A.J. (1991). Genetic contributions to human obesity. *Res Publ Assoc Res Nerv Ment Dis, 69*, 205–218.

Stunkard, A., Coll, M., Lundquist, S., & Meyers, A. (1980). Obesity and eating style. *Archives of General Psychiatry, 37*, 1127–1129.

Stunkard, A.J., Craighead, L.W., & O'Brien, R. (1980). Controlled trial of behaviour therapy, pharmacotherapy, and their combination in the treatment of obesity. *Lancet, 2*, 1045–1047.

Stunkard, A.J. & Penick, S.B. (1979). Behavior modification in the treatment of obesity. The problem of maintaining weight loss. *Archives of General Psychiatry, 36,* 801–806.

Szekely, E.A. (1988). *Never Too Thin.* The Woman's Press.

Thomason, J.A. (1983). Multidimensional assessment of locus of control and obesity. *Psychological Reports, 53,* 1083–1086.

Tiggemann, M. (1988). Gender differences in social consequences of perceived overweight in the United States and Australia. *Sex Roles,* Jan *19:1–2,* 75.

*Trimpey, J. (1989). *Rational recovery from alcoholism: The small book,* New York: Bantam.

*Trimpey, J. & Trimpey, L. (1990). *Rational recovery from fatness.* Lotus, CA: Lotus Press.

Tsujii, S., Nakai, Y., Fukata, J., & Nakaishi, S. (1988). Monoamine metabolism and its responses to food deprivation in the brain of Zucker rats. 17th annual meeting of the society for neuroscience: appetite, thirst and related disorders (1987, San Antonio, Texas). *Physiology & Behavior, 44,* 495–500.

Turner, M.S., Foggo, M., Bennie, J., & Carroll, S. (1991). Psychological, hormonal and biochemical changes following carbohydrate bingeing: a placebo controlled study in bulimia nervosa and matched controls. *Psychological Medicine, 21,* 123–133.

Van Itallie, T.B. & Lew, E.A. (1990). Health implications of overweight in the elderly. *Progress in Clinical Biological Research, 326,* 89–108.

Van, S. (1985). Eating behavior, personality traits and body mass in women. *Addictive Behaviors, 10,* 333–343.

*Velten, E. (Speaker) (1989). *How to be unhappy at work.* Cassette recording. New York: Institute for Rational-Emotive Therapy.

Verboeket van de Venne, W.P. & Westerterp, K.R. (1991). Influence of the feeding frequency on nutrient utilization in man: consequences for energy metabolism. *European Journal of Clinical Nutrition, 45,* 161–169.

Volkmar, F.R., Stunkard, A.J., Woolston, J., & Bailey, R.A. (1981). High attrition rates in commercial weight reduction programs. *Archives of Internal Medicine, 141,* 426–428.

Wadden, T.A., Sternberg, J.A., Letizia, K.A., Stunkard, A.J., &

Foster, G.D. (1989). Treatment of obesity by very low calorie diet, behavior therapy, and their combination: a five-year perspective. *International Journal of Obesity, 13 Suppl 2*, 39–46.

Wadden, T.A. & Stunkard, A.J. (1985). Social and psychological consequences of obesity. *Annals of Internal Medicine, 103*, 1062–1067.

Wadden, T.A. & Stunkard, A.J. (1987). Psychopathology and obesity. *Annals of the New York Academy of Sciences, 499*, 55–65.

Webb, W.W., Morey, L.C., Castelnuovo Tedesco, P., & Scott, H.W.,Jr. (1990). Heterogeneity of personality traits in massive obesity and outcome prediction of bariatric surgery. *International Journal of Obesity, 14*, 13–20.

Weinberg, R.S. (1984). Effects of preexisting and manipulated self-efficacy on weight loss in a self-control program. *Journal of Research in Personality, 18*, 352–358.

Whitelaw, A.G.L. (1971). The association of social class and sibling number with skinfold thickness in London schoolboys. *Human Biology*, Sep *43–3*, 420.

Widhalm, K., Zwiauer, K., & Eckharter, I. (1990). External stimulus dependence in food intake of obese adolescents: studies using a food dispenser. *Klin.Padiatr, 202*, 168–172.

Wilber J. F., (1991). Neuropeptides, appetite regulation, and human obesity. *Journal of the American Medical Association, 266*, 257–259.

Willard, M.D. (1991). Obesity: types and treatments. *American Family Physician, 43*, 2099–2108.

Williams, A., Spencer, C.P., & Edelmann, R.J. (1987). Restraint theory, locus of control and the situational analysis of binge eating. *Personality & Individual Differences, 8*, 67–74.

Williams, P.T. (1990). Weight set-point theory predicts HDL-cholesterol levels in previously obese long-distance runners. *International Journal of Obesity, 14*, 421–427.

Wilson, G. (1991). The addiction model of eating disorders: a critical analysis. *Advances in Behaviour Research & Therapy, 13*, 27–72.

Wilson, G. & Walsh, B. (1991). Eating disorders in the dsm-iv. special issue: diagnoses, dimensions, and dsm-iv: the science of classification. *Journal of Abnormal Psychology, 100*, 362–365.

Wilson, G.T. (1976). Obesity binge eating and behavior therapy: Some clinical observations. *Behavior Therapy, 7*, 700–701.

*Wolfe, J.L & Brand, E. (Eds.) (1977). *Twenty years of rational therapy*. New York: Institute for Rational-Emotive Therapy.

*Wolfe, J.L.(Speaker) (1980). *Woman—Assert yourself*. New York: Cassette recording. Institute for Rational-Emotive Therapy.

Wolkowitz, O.M., Doran, A.R., Cohen, M.R., & Cohen, R.M. (1988). Single-dose naloxone acutely reduces e₂ i⸱ ⸱. obese humans: behavioral and biochemical effects. *Biological Psychiatry, 24*, 483–487.

Woods, P.J. (1990). *Controlling your smoking*. Roanoke, VA: Scholars' Press.

Woods, S.C., Figlewicz Lattemann, D.P., Schwartz, M.W., & Porte, D.,Jr. (1990). A re-assessment of the regulation of adiposity and appetite by the brain insulin system. *International Journal of Obesity, 14 Suppl 3*, 69–73.

Wooley, S.C. & Wooley, W.W. (1985). Should Obesity be Treated at All? In A.J. Stunkard & E. Stellar (Eds.). *Eating and Its Disorders*, pp. 185–192, New York: Raven Press.

Wurtman, J.J., Wurtman, R.J., Mark, S., Tsay, W., Gilbert, W., & Growdon, J. (1985). D-Fenfluramine selectively suppresses carbohydrate snaking by obese subjects. *International Journal of Eating Disorders*, 89–99.

Wurtman, J.J. (1987). Disorders of food intake: excessive carbohydrate snack intake among a class of obese people. *Annals of the New York Academy of Sciences, 499*, 197–202.

Wurtman, J.J. (1988). Carbohydrate craving, mood changes, and obesity. symposium: serotonin in behavioral disorders (1987, Zurich, Switzerland). *Journal of Clinical Psychiatry, 49*, Suppl 37–Suppl 39.

*Yankura, J. & Dryden, W. (1990). *Doing RET: Albert Ellis in action*. New York: Springer.

Yates, W.R., Bowers, W.A., Carney, C.P., & Fulton, A.I. (1990). Is bulimia nervosa related to alcohol abuse? a personality analysis. *Annals of Clinical Psychiatry, 2,* 23–27.

Yates, W.R., Sieleni, B., Reich, J., & Brass, C. (1989). Comorbidity of bulimia nervosa and personality disorder. *Journal of Clinical Psychiatry, 50,* 57–59.

*Young, H.S. (1974). *A rational counseling primer.* New York: Institute for Rational-Emotive Therapy.

Young, L.M. & Powell, B. (1985). The effects of obesity on the clinical judgments of mental health professionals. *Journal of Health and Social Behavior, 26,* 233–246.

Zellner, D., Harner, D., & Adler, R. (1989). Effects of eating abnormalities and gender on perceptions of desirable body shape. *Journal of Abnormal Psychology, 98,* 93–96.

About the Authors

Albert Ellis, born in Pittsburgh and raised in New York City, holds a bachelor's degree from the City College of New York and M.A. and Ph.D. degrees in clinical psychology from Columbia University. He has been Adjunct Professor of Psychology at Rutgers University, Pittsburg State College, and other universities and has served as Chief Psychologist of the New Jersey State Diagnostic Center and Chief Psychologist of the New Jersey Department of Institutions and Agencies. He is the founder of rational-emotive therapy and the grandfather of cognitive-behavior therapy. He currently is President of the Institute for Rational-Emotive Therapy in New York City, has practiced psychotherapy, marriage and family therapy, as well as sex therapy, for almost fifty years and continues this practice at the Psychological Clinic of the Institute in New York. He is a Board of Advisors member of Rational Recovery Systems.

Dr. Ellis has published more than 600 articles in psychological, psychiatric, and sociological journals and anthologies and has authored or edited more than 50 books, including *How to Live With a "Neurotic," Reason and Emotion in Psychotherapy, A New Guide to Rational Living, A Guide to Personal Happiness, The Practice of*

Rational-Emotive Therapy, and *How to Stubbornly Refuse to Make Yourself Miserable About Anything—Yes, Anything!*

Dr. Michael Abrams is a licensed clinical psychologist in New York and New Jersey. He is Director of Psychological Medicine, a group of psychological centers headquartered in Hudson County, New Jersey, where he has worked with nearly 800 people with weight and eating difficulties. He also is a fellow of the Institute for Rational-Emotive Therapy in New York.

Dr. Abrams has specialized in weight and eating problems for many years, and has published several articles related to this topic. In addition to his work in this area, he has spent several years providing rational-emotive group and individual therapy to people with life-threatening illness, most notably AIDS.

Dr. Abrams is on the graduate faculty of Jersey City State College, where he teaches in the M.A. program in counseling. In addition to holding three degrees in psychology, Dr. Abrams holds degrees in history, business administration, and statistics, from the City University of New York and New York University.

Dr. Lidia Dengelegi is on the research faculty of Rutgers University's Institute for Health, Health Care Policy and Aging Research, and serves as Associate Director of Psychological Medicine. A licensed psychologist in New York and New Jersey, she leads group therapy and individual sessions for clients seeking help with weight and other problems. She completed a post-doctoral fellowship in rational-emotive therapy at the Institute for Rational-Emotive Therapy in New York.

In addition to her work as a clinical psychologist, Dr. Dengelegi performs research and has published widely in the field of health care and social psychology. Fluent in three languages, she is able to work with people who might normally have difficulty finding psychological help. She earned her Masters degree in psychology from New York University and her Ph.D. from Temple University.

Index